BEYOND FREUD

Beyond Freud

From Individual to Social Psychoanalysis

Erich Fromm
Edited by Rainer Funk

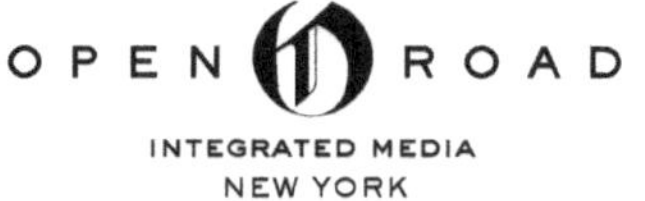

ISBN: 979-8-3372-0918-0

This edition published in 2026 by Open Road Integrated Media, Inc.
180 Maiden Lane
New York, NY 10038
www.openroadmedia.com

CONTENTS

BEYOND FREUD

I. MAN'S IMPULSE STRUCTURE AND ITS RELATION TO CULTURE

1. Psychoanalysis and the understanding of social phenomena

a) The two principles of explanation according to Freud

Social psychology is pointed in two directions. On the one hand, it deals with the problem of the extent to which the personality structure of the individual is determined by social factors and on the other hand, with the extent to which psychological factors themselves influence and alter the social process. The two sides of the problem are indissolubly bound together. The personality structure, which we can recognize as affecting the social process, is itself the product of this process and whether we observe the one side or the other, the question is only which aspect of the whole problem is the center of interest at the time.

Bearing in mind the problem of the interaction between society and the psychic structure, there is no difference in principle between social and individual psychology. Fundamentally it makes no difference whether an individual or a group is under psychological examination. The individual's manner of life is determined by society. Society itself is nothing without individuals. Freud, despite his centering of interest on the individual, recognized clearly that the difference between social psychology and individual psychology is only an apparent one.

> "Although" he says, [S. Freud, 1921c, S. E. XVIII, p. 69.], "individual psychology is carried out and concentrated on the individual, on the path he chooses to satisfy his instincts, still it happens rarely, under certain exceptional conditions, that the relationship of one to other individuals can be overlooked. In the inner life of the individual another comes up regularly as an example, as an object, as a helper and as an opponent and individual psychology therefore, is, from the beginning, also social psychology in this broader but absolutely justifiable sense".[1]

This conception is in keeping with Freud's fundamental method of explaining the psychic structure of the individual. Always fundamentally considering the influence of constitutional factors, Freud's guiding principle in the analysis of an individual is to explain the development of impulse and character structure by the experiences—especially the early childhood experiences—which the individual suffers in collision with the outside world. Put in a short formula, the principle of analytical method

1 [The foregoing verbatim quotation is Fromm's own translation. The translation of Strachey in the Standard Edition is as follows: "It is true that individual psychology is concerned with the individual man and explores the paths by which he seeks to find satisfaction for his instinctual impulses; but only rarely and under certain exceptional conditions is individual psychology in a position to disregard the relations of the individual to others. In the individual's mental life someone else is invariably involved, as a model, as an object, as a helper, as an opponent; and so from the very first individual psychology, in his extended but entirely justifiable sense of words, is at the same time social psychology as well."]

is the explanation of the impulse structure by life experiences, that is to say, the external factors that affect the individual.

Looking closer, however, it [can be] seen that this formula is too general and actually includes two different principles of explanations which are used and confused in psychoanalytical interpretation. The principle under discussion is as follows: The individual, driven by pressure for satisfaction of his needs, especially his sexual needs, must come to terms with the outside world, which serves partly as a means towards the satisfaction he seeks and partly as a hindrance to that satisfaction. In this process of adjusting to the outside world there arise certain impulses and fears, certain friendly and hostile attitudes towards the outside world, or to express it differently, [there arises] a certain type of object relation. An example of this principle of explanation is offered by the Oedipus complex.

Here Freud starts with the point that the child (for the sake of simplicity, a little boy) has sexual desires towards his mother. In attempting to fulfill the impulses corresponding to his desires he comes across his father who forbids him to satisfy these desires and threatens him with punishment. This experience with the forbidding father creates a definite psychic reaction in the child, a definite relation to the father: namely, one of hatred and hostility. The hostile impulses directed against the father meet with his superiority, which creates fear in the boy and compels him to repress these impulses: he instead submits to the father or identifies himself with him. Hostility, submission, identification are the products of the boy's collision, driven by his sexual desires, with a definite configuration in the outside world. Even aside from the question of the general validity of the Oedipus complex and of Freud's assumption that the Oedipus complex is a hereditary acquisition, the fact remains that Freud attributes the intensity and special qualities of the particular development of the Oedipus complex in an individual to the peculiarities in his life experiences.

Quite different from this principle of interpretation is one which Freud employs in explaining the connection between life experiences and the structure of drives. In this second principle, he assumes that the outside world operates on and changes sexuality in a pronounced manner, and that certain psychic impulses are the *immediate* products of specific forms of sexuality. This principle of explanation assumes the Freudian libido theory. In this theory it is assumed that sexuality goes through various developmental stages; that oral, anal, phallic and genital developmental stages are at various times centered around an erogenous zone, and further (something that more or less ties up with these erogenous zones), that certain partial sexual drives are evident, such as sadism and masochism, voyeurism and exhibitionism. Quite independent of conditions that the outside world imposes, the individual, by reason of given biological facts, goes through all these stages until matured genital sexuality becomes the dominant instinct. However, insofar as the outside world—partly through denials, partly through over-indulgence—affects the various stages of sexuality, they become fixed in one or the other form (even though such fixations, according to Freud, can be appreciately determined also by constitutional strengthening and weakening of certain erogenous zones). Thus, in contrast to normal development, they retain unusual force and become the source for development of important psychic impulses—be it through sublimation or through reaction formation. In this way Freud explains the existence of such important drives or character traits as greed, parsimony, ambition, orderliness, etc.

* * *

The foregoing analytical interpretation according to this principle also explains, in the same way, certain attitudes and certain relations to other people. Thus parsimony and greed are understood as the sublimation of the impulse to withhold the faeces. A contemptuous attitude towards people is explained by the fact that these people stand for faeces in the unconscious of an individual and the disgust he [feels] is carried over to the people. An attitude characterized by the conviction of a person that he need not exert himself at all to achieve all his ambitions, that somehow all his wishes will suddenly be fulfilled, is interpreted as the sublimation of the desire for a sudden bowel movement after a long retention of the faeces.

The difference between the two principles of explanation is obvious. In one case, a psychic phenomenon is understood to be a reaction of the individual to the outside world which has behaved in one way or another towards the fulfillment of his needs. In the other case the psychic phenomenon is directly attributed to sexuality; it is not a reaction to the outside world, but an expression of sexuality modified by the outside world.

A schematic presentation should further define this statement. The reactions falling under "I" are understood by Freud to be direct derivates of sexuality, which in turn are modified by the influences of the outside world. The reactions falling under "II" are object relations which are not the direct products of sexuality, but reactions to the outside world that occur in the process of working out the impulses.

[The following diagram is a reconstruction of an original handwritten sketch in German:]

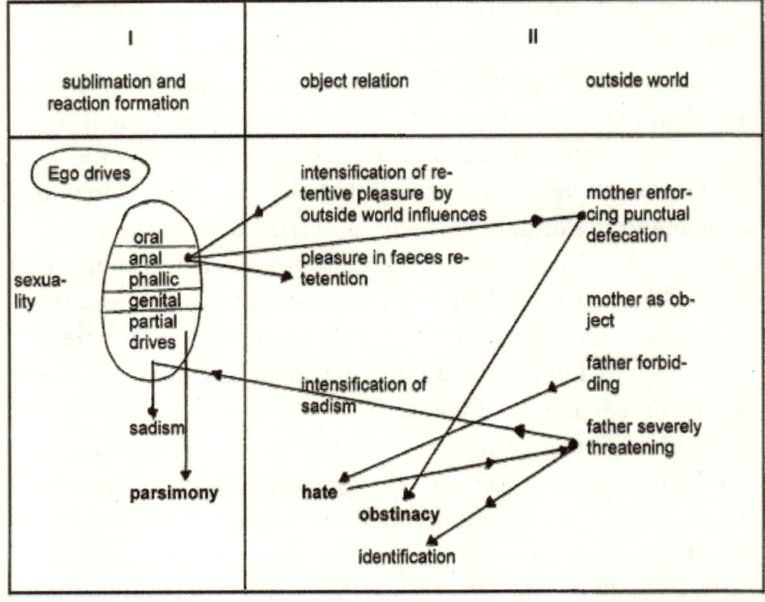

The two explanatory principles here distinguished are confused throughout psychoanalytical literature without their distinction being noted. (The differentiation between object relations and sublimation and reaction formations of genital sexuality was [recently] indicated in E. Fromm, "Die psychoanalytische Charakterologie und ihre Bedeutung für die Sozialpsychologie" ["Psychoanalytic Characterology and Its Relevance for Social Psychology"], 1932b, and at greater length by Balint.) This has led to a lack of clarity which has often [complicated] understanding the analytical theory. A good example of the confusion of the two principles of explanation is offered in the concept of the anal characters conceived by Freud and carried further by others, especially Abraham and Jones. Freud found [that] a frequently repeated syndrome of three character traits, orderliness, parsimony and [obstinacy], [was] associated with definite experiences in the history of defecation and the toilet habit. Obstinacy or wilfulness is understood to be a reaction to an outside world which confronts the infant with hostility and strictness in regard to its physiological needs. The principle of explanation here is the one we outlined above for the Oedipus complex. The anal function merely plays the role as an important [factor enforcing] a certain kind of contact with the outside world. Parsimony, on the other hand, is regarded as a direct product of anal eroticism, to be more exact, the pleasure in holding back the faeces, and the fact that specifically this pleasure is so strong is explained only by outside world influences.

We content ourselves here with the description of these two principles of explanation, but before we embark on a critical discussion of them we wish to present another disagreement with the Freudian theory that is important for the problem of social psychology.

b) Freud's bourgeois concept of man and his disinterest in the character of a society

We said above that Freud explains the structure of drives by life experiences, that is, outside influences at work on the individual. This statement must be [carefully delimited]. Actually, it holds only in so far as it deals with the explanation of individual differences in the impulse structure among individuals whom Freud observed in his practice or [elsewhere]. As long as he found differences here, such for instance as that of one patient who displayed an unusually strong fear of paternal authority; or another who, to an extraordinary degree, became the rival of everyone with whom he came in contact, he explained these peculiarities in the impulse structure (along with an indication of the possibility of constitutional strengthening) by the individual peculiarities in the life experiences of the patient. In one case he found, speaking very schematically, that the patient had a very strict father of whom he was afraid; in another case a sibling was born who was shown preference and against whom he developed an intense rivalry. But as long as Freud was not interested in the individual differences of his patients, but examined the psychic traits which were common to all patients, he gave up essentially the historical, that is to say, the social principle of explanation, and saw in these common traits "human nature", as it is physiologically and anatomically constituted. In other words, character structure, as is generally common to the society of normal people and of people observed by Freud, was not itself important to analyse; [indeed] for him the "middle-class character" was essentially identical with human nature.

We will content ourselves here with just a few important examples of this thesis. Freud regards the Oedipus complex as a fundamental mechanism of the entire inner life. We have indicated above that special modifications of the Oedipus complex are traced back to the peculiarities in life experiences; but the Oedipus complex is given modern man through heredity, or at least so Freud assumes hypothetically.

Another example of the same principle is found in Freud's conception of the psychology of woman. He assumes that because of knowledge of anatomical differences she must necessarily develop feelings of inferiority, resentment and envy of man, that is to say, of his genitals, and that feelings of inferiority in woman are necessary phenomena because of the lack of male sexual organs. "'Anatomy is Destiny', to vary a saying of Napoleon's" says Freud [1924d, S. E. XIX, p. 178]. The same principle of "absolutizing" the middle-class character is seen in Freud's view that the individual is primarily narcissistic, that is, fundamentally isolated from his fellow-beings and those alien to him. Even here he does not inquire into the social imputation of this phenomenon, but accepts the estranged person that he finds in our society as the necessary product of human nature.

In the same respect Freud goes even further in his theory of the death drive. While he, as he himself says, to his own surprise, originally more or less overlooked the role of non-sexual aggression in human inner life, he sees it now in its full implications. However, he does not trace it to social conditions, but assumes that, [in respect of] its quantity, it is biologically derived from the death drive, and that a person has only the alternative [in amalgamating death tendencies with erotic drives, of turning them destructively outwards or masochistically inwards].

We said that for Freud middle-class character is identical with human nature. This statement requires a certain delimitation. It would be more accurate to say that Freud identifies the fundaments of middle-class character with human nature, whereas he attributes certain influences that modify the biologically given impulse structure to culture. This leads us to touch briefly on the ideas Freud has on the relation of culture to impulse structure. Schematically they are somewhat as follows: Growing culture means growing repression of impulses. Cultural achievements are sublimations of impulses that are made possible only by the repression of impulses. But sublimation is a "talent" which is only sparingly scattered among people. Failure of sublimation leads to neurosis. Therefore, growing culture means not only a growing repression of impulses, but also a growing numbers of neuroses. Freud even goes so far as to mention the possibility that further growth of culture could lead to such an extent of impulse repression that people would no longer multiply. It is readily seen that here Freud has in mind Rousseau's picture of "Natural Man" for whom there are no repressions at all, and that his conception of the effect of culture on impulses is purely mechanistic, for he does not try qualitatively to tie up what is specific in impulse structure and what is specific in social organization, but, purely quantitatively, sees everything from the point of view of the degree of repression. In this theory Freud expresses not only a pessimistic attitude as opposed to a happy future for mankind, but he becomes so to speak the apologist for middle-class morals. In posing the alternative: "either sexual repression or no culture", he makes a psychological rationalization for the necessity or at least the value of middle-class morals.

Freud sees middle-class people moulded by outside pressure, which leads to repression and [which distinguished them] from "natural" people. Nevertheless, in a number of traits he sees an immediate expression of human nature—for instance, in the quantum of destruction converted outward or inward, or in the psychology of woman. With other traits he constructs out of the middle-class person the picture of a human nature that undergoes certain modifications only in middle-class society. His picture is a static and closed one, and on the strength of this picture he foretells all future possibilities of the inner development of human beings.

c) Critique on Freud's reductionism of spiritual and psychic phenomena to sexuality

Freud's assumption that the fundaments of the psychic structure of the middle-class individual are eternal characteristics of human nature is a prejudice which he shares with most middle-class psychologists (especially those upholding the theory of instincts), anthropologists and philosophers of his time. In the assumption that a large number of the most important drives and character traits are to be explained directly by sexuality in its various forms, the conception of the existence of a "human nature" is, however, as far as this aspect of Freudian interpretation is concerned, itself a presupposition of this part of the libido theory. At the same time another idea—characteristically philosophic [and typical of] the thinking of the social and intellectual strata from which Freud arose—forms the basis for his libido theory, namely that of bourgeois materialism, which explains spiritual and psychic phenomena as direct products of physical phenomena. Even though, as we have tried to show, the direct tracing of the psychic to the sexual represents only one aspect of Freud's method of interpretation, it represents such an important aspect, that we can rightly say that bourgeois materialism forms a [pivotally] important foundation for all Freudian thought. In his theory of the death drive, where he traces aggressiveness and such phenomena as sadism and masochism back to given biological facts, this way of thinking is even more pronounced.

What were the results of this assumption of a fundamentally eternal human nature in connection with directly tracing back important psychic strivings to sexual sources? In individual psychology the result was that Freud tended to overlook or to underemphasize a number of psychic phenomena in which the direct association with erogenous zones or partial drives could not be assumed even speculatively. The most impressive example in this respect is aggressiveness. In the discussion in which Freud presents his theory of the death drive, he remarks how odd it is that the significance of aggressiveness in human inner life had escaped him for so many years. In the theory of the death drive he succeeded again in tracing aggressiveness directly to an organic source: the biologically anchored death drive, and [hence] followed the same principle of explanation by which such traits as ambition, greed, parsimony etc. were explained. But while Freud himself here employed a corrective, even if in the wrong direction, it was not undertaken in the explanation of a large number of other psychic phenomena. The result was, as we shall show later, that a number of phenomena were not satisfactorily or sufficiently understood, and that others properly belonging to the picture of the psychic structure were [omitted] entirely.

The results were even more unfortunate for the psychological understanding of social phenomena. Starting from the view that human nature is fundamentally constant because it is determined by given biological conditions, it was impossible to arrive at a psychological interpretation of social and historical phenomena. Human nature seen thus was taken as the model by which social phenomena were explained. Characteristic examples of this method of psychological interpretation may be cited: War is "explained" as the "result" of human aggressive drives, revolution as the result of hatred towards the father, capitalism as the result of the extraordinarily strong anal libido in people of this epoch. Whenever alien social forms different from middle-class culture were examined, it was not deemed necessary to analyse them, [i.e., to ask]: how a certain social structure will produces a certain character structure, but instead analogies [were deemed sufficient] and an effort was made to show that certain similarities exist between the behavior of people in a society and the symptoms of neurotic individuals. The assumption was even made by inferences from analogy that the reasons for the behavior of people in another culture are the same as the reasons for neurotic behavior in patients. (Compare my polemic regarding this point against the analogy method Theodor Reik employs in his explanation of the Christ dogma in E. Fromm, 1930a.)

The psychologism in the interpretation of social phenomena necessarily led to the complete ignoring of determining social derivations of phenomena under examination or at least to the false evaluation of their importance.

This [wrong track] on which orthodox analytical interpretation of social phenomena found itself is all the more noteworthy since one of the aspects of the Freudian method of interpretation, namely understanding psychic phenomena as the product of the collision of the person seeking satisfaction of his needs with the given outside world constellation, would have led to the proper social psychological method. If the psychic impulses and the whole character structure of the individual are determined by the special form of his individual experiences, then those of the people of a society or class with *common* traits, that is, of typical character structure are determined by the common experiences of this group, that is, by their way of life; in the last analysis [this] is prescribed for them [by] one definite [fundament], that of the form of production with its respective productive forces and [that of] the resulting social structure.

2. Psychoanalytic social psychology and its relevance for psychoanalytic theory

Freud, in the analysis of the impulse structure of individuals made a method of the hitherto unknown minute examination of all the individual life experiences and individual life practice. The use of the same principle for the analysis of the character structure typical of a social group requires a correspondingly exhaustive knowledge of the whole life practice of this group, and, in turn, [requires] analysis of the fundamental economic and social conditions within the life practice. The same role the individual life history plays in the analysis of an individual is played by the economic and social structure in the analysis of the character structure of a group. The understanding of the life practice of a group is, however, a far more complex and difficult undertaking than the understanding of the life history of an individual. It presumes the analysis of the economic and social structure of this group. A knowledge of the "milieu", that is, of certain manifest social and cultural phenomena, [but] without analysis of the dynamically decisive conditions is absolutely inadequate, just as is the knowledge of single isolated economic factors, such as plenty or scarcity of food, fruitfulness or barrenness of the soil, technical development etc. Understanding of the life practice means for us analysis of the dynamics of the social structure.

The application of this method, however, leads to certain deviations from the Freudian theory, especially at those points where Freud and a number of other analysts failed in their attempt to analyse social phenomena. The most important problems from which such deviations from Freudian theory must [result] are a) the Freudian assumption that the middle-class character represents the fundamental features of human nature, b) the Freudian evaluation of the role of the family, and c) the Freudian libido theory.

a) The revision of the Oedipus complex, the concept of primary narcissism and the psychology of women

The thesis that the middle-class person with his [typical] fundamental mechanism, which Freud regards as characteristic for all human beings, is an "historical" and not a "natural" person, needs no proof here. However, for an understanding of the Freudian picture of human beings, it may be helpful to show how those traits and complexes which he regards as an inheritance of the people, are to be understood in terms of the specific present form of middle-class society. We must, however, content ourselves here too with a few indications which should clarify the underlying train of thought.

(1) The mechanism which Freud has vested with the greatest importance is the *Oedipus complex*. It consists, if we take it in its original form, and if for the sake of simplicity we orientate ourselves to the example of the little boy, of a double thesis: first, that the little boy is sexually drawn to his mother and finds her the most important object of his sexual desires; and secondly, that in doing so, he [runs up against] his father as a rival and hates him on the grounds of sexual jealousy. At the same time, because of his fear of his father and especially the fear of being "castrated", he represses his sexual wishes as well as his hostility towards his father and becomes submissive to him; that is, he identifies himself with him through the formation of the super-ego. While Freud assumes that the sexual attraction of the mother for the boy is a general human phenomenon, he believes that the repression and hostility against the father and the resulting formation of the super-ego occurred somewhere in the primitive history of mankind, but from then on belongs to the fixed heritage of human nature.

We do not wish here to go more deeply into the fact that anthropological research shows that the Oedipus complex, in Freud's sense, is not a universal complex to be found among all human beings. Nor do we wish to go into the question of whether it plays the great and general role in middle-class society ascribed to it by Freud. We [agree] that the Oedipus complex is seen in a great number of cases at any rate, and wish to ask ourselves, how it is explained by conditions specific to middle-class society.

As regards the child's sexual desires towards his mother,

there are a number of socially determined facts which explain their force. First among these is the taboo which rests upon the sexual activity of the child and especially upon sexual play with other children. We know that, among many tribes, children within the framework of their physiological development have playful sexual contact with other children, freely and without practical or moralistic interference from the outside world. In the middle-class family this natural direction of childish sexual preoccupation is blocked, for practical reasons partly and for moral reasons completely. If other children cannot be made the objects of sexual strivings then sexual desires and fantasies can be turned easily in the direction of the parents.

Certainly, this circumstance would not sufficiently explain why the taboo against sexual desires for the parent does not similarly weaken these desires if other important circumstances were not added. One of these is the fact that in middle-class society the family is the only group in which close and intimate feelings exist. Everyone not belonging to the family group is a "stranger" and stands beyond reach of the feelings of the individual and also the child. Only [those] belonging to one's own clan are loved and only from them can love be expected. This narrowing of human nearness, solidarity and love to the family group and the accompanying lack of relations to outsiders contributes to making the members of the family the most important objects of sexual desires. Freud though, in many cases, considers the intense inner relations within the family as themselves sexually determined, whereas this is hardly the case.

In his theory of the frequency and intensity of incestuous desires Freud has indeed glimpsed one of the most decisive psychic traits of middle-class society: the relatively limited expansion of feeling within the family group, which is only one side of the picture, the other being the disturbed positive feeling-relation to the "stranger". However, because of insufficient understanding of their social connotation, as when he explains all positive object relations by sexual desires, [Freud] has only been able to express these facts through theoretical distortions and, therefore, unsatisfactorily.

Another circumstance of great importance for the existence or strengthening of incestuous desires in children which, strangely enough, has been scarcely mentioned by Freud, is to be sought in the conduct of parents. While cases where the parents consciously and overtly accost their children manifestly and seduce them in one way or another are rare (to be sure, far less rare than is generally believed) [there are a great number of] cases where the father or the mother has sexual impulses towards the child which are essentially unconscious. The missing quality of awareness does not alter the fact that the impulses are there and that they have a certain seductive and stimulating effect on the child. A very close scrutiny of the conduct of the parents shows in how many ways the subtle seduction or sexual stimulation of the children is accomplished by the parents and show that many of the incestuous desires we find in children are reactions to this stimulation.

The fact that parents develop sexual desires towards their children is, however, itself founded in the social situation, specifically in the relative sexual dissatisfaction of most people [that is] a characteristic of middle-class society. In that from early childhood sexuality is covered with the stigma of the bad and the forbidden; in that the choice of a marriage partner is for the most part quite independent of mutual sexual attraction. In that extra-marital relations are factually blocked or [covered] with the stigma of the forbidden; in that the entire life practice of the middle-class individual reduces to a minimum the capacity for enjoyment and happiness, sexual as well as every other kind, a situation arises in which for an extraordinarily large number of people marriage permits only a very limited satisfaction of sexual impulses. This unsatisfied sexuality is one of the conditions that cause the child to become the object, even though largely unconsciously so, of sexual feelings.

If children's sexual desires towards their parents are to be explained to a considerable degree by the specific structure of middle-class family, then [too] the other side of the Oedipus complex, the hostile rivalry towards the other parent, is also [grounded] in the same structure. Certainly, sexual desires, as far as they exist, result in a certain degree of rivalry and hostility towards the parent of the same sex, [such] as the jealousy of the little boy towards his father. But factors of tremendous importance are quite overlooked when the degree of hostility and rivalry which is actually found in the relation of the boy to his father is understood primarily as the product of sexual jealousy.

A decidedly more important factor for the breeding of this hostility lies in the structure of the middle-class family. The situation of the child is one of the subjection to parents, especially paternal authority. The Roman *pater familias* had power of life and death over his son; in the middle-class family this power in its practical application is limited. But the basic nature of the relationship between father and son is the same. Apart from the demand for sustaining life which is guaranteed by society, the child has no claims on the parents. Even in the most solicitious and friendly attitude of parents towards the child there clings, in the middle-class family, the flavor of conferring favors. Society gives the child no claims to such an attitude, it represents a gift and no inalienable right. Actually, in the vast majority of cases, the attitude of parents is hardly one of unconditional well-wishing and deep friendliness. The child is the object of their authority, as a matter of fact the only one for most people. The parents expect satisfaction from him, whether grossly economic, or psychological and emotional. Self-will and independence in the child are broken in a more or less brutal manner during the first years of his life, his freedom and individuality repressed.

This relationship of parents and children, anchored in the structure of the middle-class family, is abetted by a number of circumstances, which are determined by the total structure of society. The helplessness and powerlessness of an individual in middle-class society, the fact that he is the object of personal and impersonal powers which determine his life, and upon which he has no influence, breed a psychic structure in which alongside the masochistic tendency to submit to others, the sadistic tendency to make the weak and the helpless objects of one's own authority plays a decisive role. The child, in this sense, is the most important object of sadistic tendencies.

Closely connected is the extraordinary degree of hostility which is engendered in the individual of a society built on the battle of one against all, [and which] necessarily finds its expression in the attitude of the parents to the child. Whether this hostility is expressed in brutal scenes or in more subtle form, whether it is frequently manifest or merely simmers as a threat which forces the child into submission is of secondary importance. Here we must add something else. A society built on the principle of individual competition brings about an attitude of permanent rivalry towards others, with which the child is imbued quite early; on the basis of this attitude there exists a permanently hostile comparison and rivalry with everyone who can play the role of rival, whether it is the brother or the sister or the father.

The views touched upon here represent an attempt to show

that the Oedipus complex, regarded by Freud as such a central phenomenon that he makes it an essential part of human nature, has its determining roots in the specific structure of the middle-class family and in middle-class society. As for the other traits which Freud attributes to "human nature," this connection is even more obvious. The extraordinary degree of hostility which Freud traces to the existence of a biologically determined death drive is permanently and necessarily engendered by the life practice of middle-class society. The assumption that it is a natural phenomenon is based on the same perpetuation of the middle-class character as the older bourgeois theory that the principle *homo homini lupus* is the fundamental principle of all social life.

(2) Freud's picture of the human being includes, along with the above mentioned trait of primally hostility and destructiveness, the assumption that the individual is *primal narcissistic.* Freud starts with the point that the individual originally loves only himself and is concerned only with himself and that all relations to objects, especially the feeling of love and solidarity with others, are secondary attitudes built on that basis, which can readily disappear, giving way to the fundamental narcissistic attitude. We cannot here enter further into the problem of Freud's confusion of two things in his conception of narcissism—self-love and the lack of friendly feelings towards [one's] fellow man. In fact, he considers all lack of friendliness as narcissistic phenomena. His assumption is that an "exchange relationship" exists, in which the more love there is for others, the less self-love there can be and *vice versa*. We, on the contrary, find that, actually, the capacity for love of others and of oneself have a common source and run parallel. Where this capacity is disturbed, a genuine friendliness exists neither towards oneself

nor towards others. Nevertheless, Freud has struck, in his idea of narcissism one of the most deep-seated and underlying traits of the middle-class person: his isolation, seclusion, his monadic character.

The middle class individual represents a self-secluded system, revolving in and around itself, in which other individuals and all things are estranged and are only the means of satisfying needs. For the first time in history, middle-class society has developed a person who has sprung the barriers of primitive blood and communion, and established himself as an individuality. At the same time, however, by separating this individual from others, it has made him into a being fundamentally antagonistic to others. We cannot here attempt to show to what extent this isolated, unfriendly person is the product of middle-class life practice, of middle-class means of production and the social structure which is built up from it. In this connection it is only necessary for us to show that the fundamental narcissistic character of people, which Freud sees as a natural attribute of people, is in reality an historically determined attribute of the middle-class person.

(3) As a last example for our train of thought we wish to mention the Freudian theory of the *psychology of woman.* In this case the relation is perhaps even clearer and simpler than in the previous examples. That woman feels inferior and frequently would prefer to be a man stands to reason and is the necessary result of her position in society. She is factually dependent upon man, and only in the last decades has she begun to achieve economic and political independence; for centuries she has been hampered in developing her human capabilities and forces, she has been limited in her activities to the narrowest family circle and to developing herself on the level of "feelings" as the only

expression of her humanness; she was to be there for love only and in Freud's generation not even the capacity to enjoy sex was conceded her. She has been degraded by society to a person of second rank and this is not altered by the ideology of the romantic reactionaries who place woman as a higher being as the true bearer of love, etc. With his assumption that woman for anatomical reasons is inferior to man, and therefore jealous of him, Freud has in reality added but one more to the many rationalizations of the position of woman in society.

b) The revision of the role family has

If for a definite society or class the character structure typical of its [members] are understood as the expression of their active and passive conformity to the entire life practice of the group, then the question arises how the evaluation of the special meaning of experiences in childhood agrees with this conception, and to what extent the Freudian conception of the function of the family requires modification. Freud has shown, and this is one of his most fruitful and significant discoveries, that the experiences of the child in his earliest years are of decisive importance in the formation of his entire impulse and character structure. Analytical experience shows that this is correct even if one differs with the Freudian conception in holding that the experiences of the child after the fifth or sixth year play a greater role in the further development of the character structure than he believes, and in not regarding the further development as a pure repetition, in a mechanical way, of the reaction [laid down] in early childhood.

Since the life of the child—and the European to a greater degree than the American—is centered, up to the sixth year, primarily around the family the special constellation in the family must appear as the reason for peculiarities in character development. As far as individual differences between personalities are concerned this is true and "reasons" (in this sense) for differences in character structure are to be found in certain differences in the family constellation. But what [are we say] of character structure in general [as it] typifies a society or class? The child hardly comes in contact with social life as such. The most important categories of social life, like money-making, desire for profit, business competition, the possibility of satisfying all desires with money, play as good as no role at all in the child's life.

Apparently there exists a contradiction between the thesis that the first years of a child's life are decisive for character development and the view that what determines character development is the social life practice. The solution of this apparent contradiction lies in the role of the family. The family itself is a product of the whole social structure, and it carries over to the child the most important features of the social life practice.

This holds true for the larger features of the family structure and the role of the child in it. The patriarchal family with a rather strong parental authority over the child is a product of a definite social constellation. The role of paternal authority in the family, the degree to which the child is dependent upon this authority and must submit to it, the means employed in achieving this submission, may depend upon the individual peculiarities of the parents, to a certain extent, but essentially they rest upon the entire dependence—and authority-relation within the society or class.

A society built upon the power of one class over another produces a family structure in which the same authority relation is reproduced in the relation of parents to children. This means not only that the reason for the special structure of the family is to be found in the social structure, but also that the child is familiarized in the family with the relations he will find later in social practice. The familiarizing is not of the nature of superficial "habit formation," but forms the impulse structure so that he can fulfil his later social function without friction and as prescribed by the point of view of the society to which he belongs. If it is correct to say that the psychic structure of the adult is determined by his past, by his childhood experiences, then it is equally correct to formulate the matter the other way round: the past is determined by the future, namely, by the future role of the individual, as it is stipulated by his position within his society.

The experiences of the child in the family are, however, determined by the social situation not only with regard to the fundamental structure of the family and the child's dependence upon the parents, but beyond that by the entire atmosphere the child finds in the family. The character of the parents—again in its larger features and not with regard to individual differences—is implanted by society and more specifically by the particular class to which they belong. As parents they are not different from what they are otherwise in life. The child finds his parent's character traits as the first and most important forms of [human] expression and he reacts to them so [as to produce] corresponding character traits in him. It makes no difference whether the father faces his inferiors "as the superior" or whether "as a father", he makes the child his helpless tool and insists upon unconditional submission. Whether as in the first case, the rationalizations are very thin or fail altogether or, as in the second case, the father is convinced that everything he does is for the good of the child—what the child experiences depends not upon the rationalizations but upon the behavior of the father. The child has, as yet, little sensitivity to rationalizations: the young child would not even understand them if expressed in words. A commanding gesture, a sadistic gleam in the eye and the threatening tone of voice are, even by the very small child, fully understood; usually better than by the grown-up, who has become accustomed to taking seriously only what is verbally expressed.

We cannot here attempt to show how all the underlying traits and characteristic of the members of a society or of a class find their expression in the behavior of parents towards their children. It is sufficient that we have shown what is essential: that what the child in the family experiences is the reflection of the life of the society, that the family is not the "reason" for the formation of character but represents the mechanism for transmission of socially given traits to the individual. Expressed differently, the *family is the psychological agent of society*. The study of the family structure is indispensable for the understanding of a personality structure typical of a society, for only the knowledge of the details of family life and the method of rearing children can give an insight into how social exigencies, insofar as they concern the personality, [are transposed] into the individual psyche. [In regard to] the analysis of society, [I consider it inappropriate] to rest content with a presentation of its educational process. The educational process itself must be analysed in the light of its social circumstances.

Among the anthropologists, particularly Margaret Mead in her various works: *Coming of Age in Samoa* [1928], *Growing up in New Guinea* [1929], *Sex and Temperament* [1935, William Morrow & Company, New York], has pointed to the significance of childhood for the development of the personality structure. This represents, without question, an important step forward. Our criticism here too, however, would be that the particular kind of educational process cannot be construed as the final principle of explanation.

c) The revision of the theory of drives according to a different concept of man

More important and more fundamental than the two deviations from the Freudian theory discussed till now, is the further deviation [with reference to] the Libido theory [. . .]. It concerns a part of the theory that is regarded by many analysts and non-analysts as so fundamental that the following views may no [longer] be regarded as "psychoanalytical." We do not believe this, but, quite to the contrary, feel that they are a consistent continuation of the Freudian method, dictated by necessity if Freud's philosophical assumptions, especially his physiological materialism, are set aside; and if at the same time the life practice of people is seen in its decisive role, beyond the narrow framework of individual differences.

We said at the beginning of this paper that Freud uses [and confused] two methods of interpretation [. . .]. One holds that psychic impulses, fears, behavior and the resulting character traits are to be understood as the reaction of the individual to a definite outside-world constellation which he comes across in the process of carrying out his needs. The other method of interpretation is to understand important psychic impulses and character traits as only another "physical state" of sexual needs themselves, modified in a specific way by influences from the outside world but [still in their] fundamentals physiologically given entities. We believe that Freud's first method must be consistently continued and developed into a general principle of explanation for all psychic impulses and behavior, with the exception of course, of impulses such as sexuality, hunger thirst, etc. which require no psychological explanation but a physiological one. However, the assumption that impulses like parsimony, greed, orderliness, etc. can be understood as direct offshoots of sexual strivings, more correctly, of the pregenital libido, seems to us untenable.

The most cogent [reasons for] this assumption have been my experiences in psychoanalysis. The Freudian libido theory was a theoretical supposition on the strength of which these experiences were gathered. But despite very intensive efforts to arrive at an understanding of character as a sublimation or reaction formation of pregenital sexuality, the efforts seemed more and more hopeless. Certainly, in some cases, it could be seen that in persons who were irrationally parsimonious, ambitious or orderly, the entire defecation history had a significance beyond the average degree. But attempting to "interpret" parsimony as a sublimation of pleasure in withholding the faeces usually resulted not only in no change in behavior, but also no great deepening of the understanding of the phenomenon. Even if it could be assumed or guessed that the pleasure in holding back the faeces was developed early on the grounds of defiant outside influences, the basis for explaining a trait as significant for the entire personality as parsimony was extremely small; furthermore, this explanation was incapable of encompassing the trait in its connection with the whole personality structure and as an expression of it. In many other cases there was no such connection at all. A strong, driving parsimony was found, but early childhood experiences in regard to bowel movements were absolutely normal. In other cases it could be seen that a certain pleasure in retarding the bowel movement may have existed in fact, but when the amount of this pleasure was compared with that in other cases where no greed developed, the quantitative difference seemed in no wise commensurate with the assumed end result in character of early childhood experiences. The same observation held not only for attributes of the anal character, but even more for attributes such as ambition, whose alleged causal connection with urethral eroticism almost never appeared, even as a vague speculation. We shall return before [long] to the question as to how far the connection occasionally found between the special interest in defecation and character traits such as greed can be explained without drawing upon anal eroticism as the source of or reason for greed.[2]

Next in importance to clinico-analytical experiences were sociological and social-psychological deliberations which led to the task of examining that part of Freud's libido theory here under question. Thus, for instance, character traits designated by Freud as anal are found to a pronounced and, in relation to the rest of society, to a markedly greater degree in the European lower middle-classes. According to Freud's theory, the assumption would have to be made that prevalence of the anal character structure in the European lower middle-classes stems either from a special constitutionally determined excitation of the anal zone, or that certain experiences in toilet training are common to all lower middle-class people, which are responsible for the pleasure in withholding the faeces or the fixation on the anal level.

---

2 The question of what role the therapeutic success of an analysis plays as proof of the validity of a theory is very complicated. On the one hand, there is no doubt that a therapeutic success in itself proves nothing about the validity of a theory. Experiments with all kinds of open or veiled suggestion therapy show that there is almost no method with which therapeutic success cannot be attained. If a therapeutic success can be attained with an interpretation that is theoretically wrong then it plays the same role as any other method of suggestion. The patient is told: "This and that are the reasons for your symptoms, and after we have found them, the symptoms must disappear." As suggestion, the same effect can be achieved by telling him: "The reason for your symptom lies in an angry spirit, which we must drive out." But, on the other hand, the point of view that therapeutic success in itself says nothing for the validity of the theory should not lead us to severance of the connection between theory and therapeutic effectiveness and to fail to put the question as to whether an interpretation helps or not. In what sense therapeutic success can be considered as a criterion for the theoretical validity of an interpretation is an extremely complicated problem. One thing, however, can be said: Therapeutic success by no means proves anything about the validity of a theory, but the failure of therapeutic effectiveness in every instance of interpretation must at least perplex the analyst and compel him to re-test his theory.

Certainly, even according to Freud, the repression of genital sexuality, which actually occurs in the lower middle-classes to a greater degree than in other social classes, would be an essential condition for the regression to the anal level. But even allowing this factor, the basis of explanation remains very meager, especially if it is considered that, on the one hand, greed is only [one factor in] a character structure which, in its entirety, can only be explained as "anal" if the point is forced. On the other hand, the whole life practice of this class permits a much more satisfactory explanation of this structure.

The lack of relation between assumed reason and characterological effect becomes even clearer in a character trait such as ambition, which is socially one of the most relevant traits of the middle-class person. If, in the matter of anal eroticism, the possibility of certain common experiences in toilet training together with sexual repression leading to certain characterological results can still be entertained, then the further assumption that something in the structure of middle-class society must be [responsible for] the singularity of urethral eroticism—that the intensity of ambition, which is so characteristic of the middle-class person, must have its roots in the peculiarities of urethral eroticism—is a grotesque speculation.

To these objections arising from empirical deliberations, purely theoretical ones may be added. They concern the principal suppositions of the Freudian libido theory. Freud, as far as his theory relates to psychic impulses as direct derivatives of pregenital sexuality, is an instinct theoretician, and the theoretical deliberations and goals of such a theoretician have led him to that part of his theoretical construction where he conceives the psychic as the direct derivate of pregenital sexuality, [. . .] i.e. the direct product of an instinct. Certainly, his libido theory, in spite of its apparent primitiveness, represents an enormous step beyond the instinct theories. While these, essentially, hypostasize "behavior" and assume an inborn instinct behind all important behavior, Freud saw the "structuralness" of the psychic apparatus, discovered that the driving forces are unconscious and recognized the mechanisms in which the unconscious forces push their way through to consciousness or express themselves in behavior.

In the great literature that came into being as a reaction to the instinct theories, especially since 1919, this has been so thoroughly criticised that we can be satisfied at this time merely with mentioning the literature.[3]

We wish here only to go into one point, which is not stressed there. The instinct theories tend towards basing human psychology in drives psychology; they overlook the fact that just as the individual has created a second nature in his implements, so too a second nature [has been created] psychologically [in the form of those] very psychic impulses and behavior that are specific to the individual and are themselves neither inborn nor physically founded instincts nor their direct derivatives. The instinct theories from [Wilhelm Thierry] Preyer on developed in reference to the Darwinian theory. They show, for the realm of psychology, that the human being—despite of all religious and idealistic assumptions—is determined like the animal by inborn impulses founded in the physical organism. This use of the theory of evolution in psychology certainly meant an enormous stride. But in stressing the psychological factors common to man and animal, the decisive differences

3 The following are named as the most important anti-instinctivistic [standpoints]: K. Dunlap, 1929; Z. Y. Kuo, 1921 and 1922; the extremely thorough and instructive book of the sociologist L. L. Bernard *Instincts* (1924) and Dewey's *Human Nature and Conduct* (1922), which takes an intermediary position. G. Murphy (1932) gives a short and excellent view of the instinct theory.

between man and animal and the fact that man has developed qualities not found in the animal kingdom were overlooked. This is no objection to the evolutionary finding that man developed from the animal, but only to the mechanistic theory of evolution which does not recognize that quantitative changes are converted into new qualities, those specific to human beings.

In social and economic respects the qualitative difference between animal and human existence is expressed, above all, in the fact that the human being produces and the animal does not. By production we mean active alteration of natural surroundings, going beyond pure gathering, and the creation of new elements by simple combinations of existing ones. The symbols of production in this sense are fire and implements. The point in animal and human existence where quantity was converted into quality would be where the human being made a fire for the first time and used implements, however primitive.

The same view can be expressed from another angle. The animal's adjustment to its surroundings is, essentially, purely passive, the human being's passive and at the same time active. Darwin has shown that the development of the physiological and anatomical structure of animals and humans is to be understood in the sense of a process of adjustment to surrounding conditions. The animal remains in this state of passive adjustment and his relation to the surroundings is, in principle, static. The human being after he ceased to develop anatomically and physiologically began an active process of adjustment. He actively changes his surrounding conditions and in this process is himself changed: no longer anatomically and physiologically, but, primarily, psychologically. His relation to nature undergoes permanent transformation. The same state of affairs may be expressed in still another way: man has a history, animal is without history.[4]

What is the psychological aspect of this matter? The relation of the animal to his surroundings, the manner in which it comes to terms with and overcomes them is essentially laid down in heredity. Despite the presence of certain possibilities of modification in the manner of encountering the environment, which grow as we ascend the hierarchy of the animal kingdom, it is essentially correct to say that the inherited reflexes and instincts regulate the relation of the animal to his surroundings and that the manner of this relation to, and of coming to terms with, the surroundings is for every subhuman species relatively fixed and unchanging.

In the human being the means of coming to terms with nature is no longer hereditarily fixed. His adjustment to the surroundings does not occur in biological periods but in historical ones, and in this process of adjustment he changes the surroundings as well as himself. Only the fact that the fixed hereditary manner of facing the environment was loosened or [suspended] in human beings, created the possibility of a history and culture.

Man, like the animal, has a number of drives founded in his physical organism, of which we wish to mention the most important and undisputed: hunger, thirst and sexuality. The goal of these physiological drives is the outlet of tensions produced by physical and especially internal chemical sources. These physiological drives are the ones, in the last analysis, which drive the human being as well as the animal to "live," that is, to come to grips with the human and non-human surroundings for the purpose of satisfying these needs. But the manner of doing so

4 The point of view defended here on the fundamental difference between animal and human development was also aroused by C. J. Warden, 1936.

is not fixed in human beings by contrast with lower animals. The only condition that is common to all people is that they can only produce as social beings, that is, not only the satisfaction of sexuality but all the need to maintain life demands that the human being enter into social relations with others.

The form in which the individual can satisfy his sexual needs and maintain his existence is prescribed by certain objective conditions. These conditions consist in what the natural surroundings [at any given time offers] a society by way of consumption goods, and the degree of power man has over nature—or, expressed differently, in the development of the productive forces. The form of production depends upon this, and this in turn determines the person's way of life which again determines the psychic structure of the person, the kind of relations to other people, the specific impulses and fears which arise, as a result of a particular form of satisfying his needs. While the physiological needs are basically the same for all and while they are the immediate products of the human organism, the psychic impulses are produced as reactions by the individual to the previously determined conditions under which he can satisfy his physiological needs. *Thus we arrive at two elements in the psychic structure which must be differentiated: the naturally given physiological drives and the historical psychic impulses, developed in the social process. These form the object of human psychology.*

People differ psychologically, not in the fact that they have hunger, thirst and sex needs, but in the particular kind of psychic structure they have, and this psychic structure develops as a historical product. The most important elements of the psychic structure are the attitude of the individual to others or to himself, or, as we should like to say, the basic human relation, and the fears and impulses which, in part directly, in part indirectly, arise out of this behavior. The basic human relation can be the original unity that we find among many primitive tribes, as it appears before the emergence of people as individualities different from one another. It can be a monadic isolation and seclusion of one individual from another, as is characteristic of middle-class society, and it can be active union and solidarity on the basis of the emergence of human individuality, that is to say, a solidarity that is fundamentally different from the pre-individual first level. Here the most important psychic impulses, as far as the forms of relations to people are concerned, are destructiveness, love and sado-masochism; as far as the forms of consumption goods [are concerned] they are the impulses to receive passively, to take forcibly, to save and to produce. Fears typical of a certain character structure are determined by the contents of the needs which are predominantly important in this psychic impulse structure and the degree of threat by a given outside world constellation. From these fundamental attitudes, impulses and fears a vast number of complex impulses and attitudes are built.

3. The difference in psychoanalytic theory illustrated on the anal character

a) It is not only a matter of sexuality and its derivates

What is the essential difference between the impulse theory here presented and the Freudian theory? As far as one side of the Freudian method is concerned, namely explaining the psychic structure as a reaction to the behavior of the outside world towards the individual, we essentially follow Freud's method. Like Freud, we start from the point that the person is primarily driven by certain physiologically anchored needs, and like him we understand psychic impulses as a reaction to the behavior of the outside world towards satisfaction of these impulses. A difference exists here insofar as for us, among the needs the person is driven by, the sexual ones do not play the same dominant role as for Freud. Then comes, as in principle also in Freud, the need for self-preservation. But in the course of historical development this is joined by other needs, some psychic—historical in the sense expounded above—like sado-masochistic impulses or the impulse to save, etc., whose experiences in coming to terms with other people again call forth new reactions and finally, the physiologically determined needs for the preservation of life [are joined by] come the socially determined, like the need for richer and more varied food, living quarters, etc., and the entire domain of needs for new material wealth, as these are created in [the course of] historical development.

The decisive difference from the Freudian libido theory lies then in the way of explaining those impulses which Freud regards as direct derivatives of sexuality and especially pregenital sexuality and the partial impulses. We believe that these too, directly or indirectly, find their explanation in object relations, not in the outflow of instincts; that impulses are [involved], which come about in the individual as reactions to the outside world and in an outside world in which he must satisfy his needs in a certain, definite way. The psychic structure of the person, as far as it goes beyond given physiological needs common to all people, is understood from the person's way of life, from his activity or from the specific forms of his life process, and not as the direct product of the physiological impulses themselves; *his life process, in which the physiological needs are but an aspect, and not his physiology, forms the material basis by which his psychic structure can be understood.*

b) Freud's description and interpretation of the anal character

We wish to illustrate our point with the example of the interpretation of the anal character. In a treatise published in 1908 on "Character and Anal-eroticism" Freud says: "Among the persons one sought to help with psychoanalysis, a type very frequently met with is very excellent because of the combination of certain character traits, while the behavior of a certain body function and the organs involved in the childhood of these persons drew attention to themselves."[5] The character traits Freud found in frequent combination were, orderliness, parsimony and wilfulness. The body function that drew attention to itself because of its behavior [was that of] bowel movement.

This syndrome of character attributes observed by Freud covers a series of character traits related to one another. "'Orderliness' encompasses bodily cleanliness as well as also conscientiousness in small duty fulfillments and dependability; the opposite of this would be: 'lack of orderliness,' 'carelessness.' Parsimony can appear aggravated to greed; wilfulness becomes obstinacy with a tendency to rage and thirst for revenge tying up to it. The two last traits—parsimony and wilfulness—are more closely related to each other than to the first, "orderliness"; they are also a more constant part of the whole complex, though it seems to me undeniable that somehow all three belong together."[6]

5 [The translation of Strachey in the Standard Edition is as follows: "Among those whom we try to help by our psycho-analytic efforts we often come across a type of person who is marked by the possession of a certain set of character-traits, while at the same time our attention is drawn to the behavior in his childhood of one of his bodily functions and the organ concerned in it." (S. Freud, 1908b, S. E. IX, p. 169.)]

6 ["'Orderly' covers the notion of bodily cleanliness, as well as of conscientiousness in carrying out small duties and trustworthiness. Its opposite would be 'untidy' and

The clinical observation Freud made regarding the intestinal function was that persons in whom this character syndrome was found, "required a relatively long time before they mastered infantile *incontinentia alvi*, and that even in later childhood complained of single failures in this function. They seem to have belonged to those infants who rebel against moving their bowels when placed on a pot, because they get incidental pleasure out of defecation: they admit that even in somewhat later years it gave them pleasure to hold back the stool and recall, even if sooner and more readily about their brothers and sisters than about themselves, all kinds of unseemly preoccupations with the faeces they produced."[7]

The observation of the simultaneous appearance of that trio of character traits and the described peculiarities in these people's experiences of toilet training led Freud to the theoretical conclusion that both facts are causally related. He assumes that in childhood the erogenous emphasis on the anus zone was especially marked; "but since after the passing of childhood these weaknesses and peculiarities can no longer be found in these people, we must assume that the anal zone lost its erogenous significance, in the course of development and presume then that the constancy of that trio of attributes in

---

'neglectful'. Parsimony may appear in the exaggerated form of avarice; the obstinacy can go over into defiance, to which rage and revengefulness are easily joined. The two latter qualities—parsimony and obstinacy—are linked with each other more closely than they are with the first—with orderliness. They are, also, the more constant element of the whole complex. Yet it seems to me incontestable that all three in some way belong together." (S. Freud, 1908b, S. E. IX, p. 169.)]

7 [The text according to Strachey's translation: ". . .that they took a comparatively long time to overcome their infantile *incontinentia alvi*, and that even in later childhood they suffered from isolated failures of this function. As infants, they seem to have belonged to the class who refuse to empty their bowels when they are put on the pot because they derive a subsidiary pleasure from defecating; for they tell us that even in somewhat later years they enjoyed holding back their stool, and they remember—though more readily about their brothers and sisters than about themselves—doing all sorts of unseemly things with the faeces that had been passed." (S. Freud, 1908b, S. E. IX, p. 170.)]

their character must be connected with the dissipation of anal eroticism".[8]

To clarify this theoretical assumption Freud reaches back to the presentation he made in *Drei Abhandlungen zur Sexualtheorie ["Three Essays on the Theory of Sexuality"]*. There he tried to show that excitations come from the so-called erogenous zones (genitals, mouth, anus, urethra) which he comprehended as "sexual excitations." While originally the excitations in these parts of the body arise directly and physically, in the course of development an essential part of those sexual excitations becomes diverted from the original sexual goal and is "sublimated". The assumption lay at hand that we "recognize in the character attributes so frequent in former anal erotics—orderliness, parsimony and wilfulness—as the first and most constant results of sublimation of anal eroticism."[9] At the end of this treatise, of only eight pages, Freud indicates the expectation that "also other character complexes can be recognized as belonging to the excitations of certain erogenous zones."[10]

He sums up his perception of the impulses lying at the root of

8 [Strachey's translation is the following: "But since none of these weaknesses and idiosyncrasies are to be found in them once their childhood has been passed, we must conclude that the anal zone hat lost its erotogenic significance in the course of development; and it is to be suspected that the regularity with which this triad of properties is present in their character may be brought into relation with the disappearance of their anal erotism." (S. Freud, 1908b, S. E. IX, p. 170.) He sums up his perception of the impulses lying at the root of character formation in the following formula: "The remaining character traits are either unchanged continuations of the original impulses, sublimation of the same, or reaction formations to the same." [Strachey's translation: "The permanent character-traits are either unchanged prolongations of the original instincts, or sublimations of those instincts, or reaction-formations against them." (S. Freud, 1908b, S. E. IX, p. 175.)]

9 [Strachey translates as follows: "It is therefore plausible to suppose that these character-traits of orderliness, parsimony and obstinacy, which are so often prominent in people who were formerly anal erotics, are to be regarded as the first and most constant results of the sublimation of anal erotism." (S. Freud, 1908b, S. E. IX, p. 171.)]

10 [Strachey's translation: "We ought in general to consider whether other character-complexes, too, do not exhibit a connection with the excitations of particular erotogenic zones." (S. Freud, 1908b, S. E. IX, p. 175.)]

character formation in the following formula: “The remaining character traits are either unchanged continuations of the original impulses, sublimation of the same, or reaction formations to the same.”[11]

Freud’s hypothesis presented here was taken over completely by the psychoanalytical school and enlarged upon in the most varied directions without anything fundamental being changed. A number of authors, especially Abraham, Jones, Sadger, Ophuysen and Ferenczi have enlarged upon and supplemented the Freudian position to such an extent that tracing back character traits or behavior to their oral or anal source seems to belong to the iron-clad stock of psychoanalytical theory, and has become popular even far beyond the narrow circle of psychoanalysis proper.

We have already indicated above that in the Freudian interpretation of anal character two methods are actually confused, that attributes such as wilfulness are understood to be reactions to the outside world, i.e. to be object relations, and that here “anal” only plays the role of being the medium in which the interference of the outside world with the child, and his reaction to the outside world, is expressed. Parsimony, on the other hand, is regarded as a direct, even if sublimated, product of pregenital sexuality, namely the pleasure in holding back the faeces.

Freud’s apprehension of the syndrome of anal character was a fruitful and important discovery. But the question is whether the unity of the syndrome is to be traced to the uniformity of a particular erogenous zone, to which it owes its existence, or whether, as we suggest, it goes back to the uniformity of a

11 [Strachey’s translation: “The permanent character-traits are either unchanged prolongations of the original instincts, or sublimations of those instincts, or reaction-formations against them.” (S. Freud, 1908b, S. E. IX, p. 175.)]

certain way of life constellation in which the person grows up and develops in regard to certain behavior and certain impulses, namely the syndrome of the "anal character."

c) The anal character as the outcome of being related to the outside world

If we study the basic human relation, the fundamental manner of behavior towards the outside world, as we find it in people with the anal character syndrome, we find, schematically sketched, the following picture: Individuals are involved who from earliest childhood on sensed the world to be hostile, threatening and overpowering. They are not friendly towards people and the world, but secluded and isolated. They have drawn a wall around themselves behind which they have fortified themselves. Once this isolated person fortified against the world has taken this position, his "strategy" in the battle of life necessarily depends upon the strengthening and permanent entrenchment of this isolated and fortified position. Everything that can possibly serve to strengthen the wall and further entrench his position is striven for. Everything that might endanger or lift his isolation, is feared as a danger, and rightly so according to his position. Love, devotion, passion with a centrifugal direction, leading outward, are dangerous and threatening. Absolutely everything that weakens his isolated system in letting out anything is felt to be a threat, while his [security] depends upon taking into this system as much as he possibly can from the outside world.

In contrast to character types such as those Freud calls oral, that always expects to receive something from the world, or sadistic, that exploits other people and wants to take things away from them, the anal character is still further advanced in his isolation and withdrawal from the outside world. He does not hope for a friendly outside world that will give him something, whether by submitting to it, or by making himself liked; on the other hand, he feels himself too weak to exploit others and take something from them. If he does not expect to receive anything from others, and has at the same time a deep feeling to produce and to achieve his desires, then for him only one way is left to reassure himself in the world and acquire a maximum in treasures, namely, to use up nothing and to hoard everything once it enters into his system. The special position of his relation to other people fosters this tendency tremendously. Every one is a potential enemy who wishes to get something from him, and he must always protect himself against this danger. On the grounds of this basic attitude towards the world and towards himself, that is, his isolation, his feeling of weakness, his latent hostility and fear of other people's hostility, the impulse to save is developed as the dominating form of acquisitiveness or of [securing] his person in regard to his material needs.

The impulse to save, in the sense in which Freud and myself are speaking of, means something emotional, something driving. It does not involve a rational attitude, made necessary by externally given facts, but an emotional, irrational drive that makes saving a necessity, [deriving] from somewhere within, regardless whether the external circumstances demand it or not. An extreme example of purely irrational parsimony is seen in those pathological cases of greed, where wealthy people deny themselves every joy and their only pleasure consists in piling up money and objects. Less extreme cases are those people who cannot part with anything and must collect everything even if it represents no material value. But it is clear that parsimony in the emotional, irrational sense becomes extremely intensified when it is also, at the same time, determined by the actual life situation and is factually under the given circumstances the prescribed attitude.

It is often difficult to discover whether in certain people only the externally conditioned attitude is involved or whether parsimony in this psychological sense. As far as observing this attitude [is concerned,] it is most clearly defined in the following directions. Where irrational parsimony exists it is found that people are parsimonious not only regarding objects of material worth but also regarding things of no value whatsoever, such as old newspapers or used shoelaces; further, that they are also parsimonious in regard to every thing else besides objects, for instance with feelings or memories. (One of the unconscious motives of sentimentality may be connected with a sort of pleasure in collecting memories of past experiences.) It is further found that these people, even if their material circumstances change—if they become either so rich that saving is no longer necessary or so poor that saving no longer pays—continue their parsimonious attitude with the same intensity.

Where parsimony exists in close relation to the practical circumstances the relation of wilfulness or orderliness to the practical circumstances is much looser. They both grow out of the same basic relationship to the world, out of which parsimony in its irrational aspects stems. Wilfulness is the tendency to self-assertion, on the basis of the feeling of the world's hostility and the concomitant lack of strength to overcome it or to assert oneself against it. Wilfulness wants to defend the constantly threatened, isolated system "I" against an overpowering world and does it by stressing or overstressing every peculiarity, every small bit of singularity in this "I." The wilful person refuses to win people or gain things either in hostile or in friendly and productive ways. He is only concerned with permitting no entrance from the outside into his system, he is compulsively and convulsively on the defensive. Precisely because he feels weak and incapable of offensive in decisive matters, he must turn every little thing into an object of battle and demonstrate upon these little things that he is independent and not to be downed.

Orderliness—again in its irrational aspects, that is, if it goes beyond all due necessity and has an impulsive character—is closely related to wilfulness. The position of defending the person against a constantly pressing hostile world, the fear of being overrun by this world, compels, so to speak, the constant delimitation of the self-created boundaries, and thus to protect the "I" from the invasion of the world so that everything outside the "I" is always in its right place and hence can be controlled. All disorder means the danger of being overrun. Orderliness tries mechanically to avoid this danger by the constant demarcation and keeping in check of the outside world. In regard to this, the gestures of the "anal character" are very characteristic. They are all somewhat rigid and guarded, always restricted towards themselves as well as the world, in contrast to the fluid gestures of the character capable of love and drawn to the world.

In analytical literature still another trait, which in pathological cases can be especially well observed, is included under the idea of "orderliness," namely, irrational cleanliness or its pathological form of expression, the compulsion to wash. Abraham and others consider this trait to be a reaction formation to still existent unconscious pleasure in playing with faeces. We believe that it is an expression of the specific relation of this character type to the outside world. It is, like orderliness, the reaction to an untrusting, fearful basic attitude which regards the world as hostile. Every physical contact with the outside world is therefore regarded as dangerous and the stronger the fear, the stronger also the tendency is to avoid contact with the outside world. It can also happen that the outside world or especially other people are looked upon as hostile and therefore dangerous, or that certain things are taboo and therefore contact with them dangerous. Usually both go together, because the fear of taboos is itself already a product of an intensified fear of people. In washing, the dangerous contact with the outside world is removed symbolically, in a subjective way real only in the unconscious. Cleanliness in this sense is another attempt to re-erect the isolated system of the self in its purity, and to undo the contact with the outside world. It is the expression of a deep fear of and hostility towards the world.[12]

Abraham and others have supplemented Freud's originally discovered syndrome with a number of other traits, which are usually just as typical of the anal character. To these belongs, above all others, sadism. While Freud saw in sadism a partial drive of sexuality (now a mixture of sexuality and the death drive), which was never clearly connected with anal eroticism, we believe that it is an expression of the same fundamental attitude and object relation, that lies at the roots of the "anal character."

By sadism we mean the drive to make another person or some creature a meek tool of one's own power, like "putty in one's hands." The particular form of sadism that forces the other person to endure physical tortures is only an extreme expression of this tendency, for there is no greater power over another person than torture: to make him suffer and force him to cry out in pain. Sadism is always tied up with masochism and Freud has from the beginning stressed this. Originally he inclined to regard masochism as secondary, as sadism turned inward; in connection with the development of the death drive

12 [In many religions washing has quite the same function of removing a forbidden contact, whether with an unclean thing or with a member of a caste or group looked upon as dangerous or harmful.]

theory he assumed masochism to be, like sadism, primarily impulse excitations determined by the death drive. We believe that masochism too must be understood as a definite form of object relation. The masochistic tendency involves submitting to a power outside the individual conceived as overwhelmingly strong—whether another person or nature or God or the State or the past—and dissolving one's individual self in it. Here too, as in sadism, the impulse to be beaten, oppressed and humiliated, as is found in masochistic perversion or in masochistic fantasies is only an extreme expression of this general tendency.

Both sadism and masochism spring from the same human basic relation which we wish to designate as "symbiotic." We mean a relation characterized by the fact that a person in a psychic sense cannot exist alone, that he needs another to complement his own person, or better, to be the constant nutrition without which he cannot live. In masochism the accent falls on being, so to speak, swallowed by the other and in that way becoming part of him, in sadism on swallowing him and making him a part of oneself.

The sadist looks for a helpless object that he can tyrannize over boundlessly, that he can incorporate into his tyrannous purpose. The masochist looks for a powerful object to whom he can surrender himself, by whom he can be swallowed, not so much to be annihilated as to be taken up by the powerful one and become part of him. Although sadism often resembles hatred or destructiveness and masochism love, they are fundamentally different. Destructiveness wants to destroy an object, sadism to keep it and rule it; love wants to make the object happy and give to him, masochism to dissolve in him and only extinguish the self.

The symbiotic basic relation expressed in sadistic and masochistic tendencies is an aspect of the same psychic structure presented above as the basis of other "anal" character traits, namely his isolated, monadic structure with a concomitant weakness of the Ego.

d) Different explanations of character genesis and their relevance for character typologies

What about Freud's assumption that a connection exists between pregenital sexuality and character traits belonging to a certain libido level? The conception here suggested does not deny such a connection in many cases, but only sees it in a theoretically different way. The connection is seen as having two directions.

In the life of the small child toilet training represents one of the most important fields in which it collides with the outside world. The degree of denial, repression, hostility, friendliness, etc. is expressed in the medium of the regulation of the child's primitive physical functions. If parents have a repressive, hostile attitude towards the child then it will become especially defined in the manner in which the toilet habit is taught, because in spheres that play a role in the life of the adult influence on the small child does not yet come into question, and because primitive physical occurrences like defecation—or feeding—take on a more central role in the life of the small child than in adults. But it must be borne in mind that the attitude of the outside world towards the child, leading to reactions of obstinacy in the child, is not only and not necessarily connected with toilet training and in many cases there is no relation to it whatsoever. In the case of the mother whose attitude in matter of toilet training is domineering and authoritative, these traits will be present in her entire relation to the child, and this will also have the same effect upon the child if for one reason or another toilet training produces no special conflicts. If the child senses an outside world that wants to break its slowly developing will power and force it into submission, it will develop wilfulness whether the attitude of the outside world is expressed in regulating the child's toilet habits too strictly or in intimidating the child if it shows other signs of independence. Quite the same holds true for oral character traits. Freud assumes that the impulse to receive purely passively goes back to the pleasure in nursing at the mother's breast and that the particular experiences the child has in this connection are determining in the development of this pleasure. Here too, we find adequate numbers of cases where a person developed this attitude of receiving passively already early in childhood, however, not because anything unusual happened in his childhood experiences in regard to feeding, but because the attitude of the outside world towards the child was overdenying and intimidating or overprotective, [thus inhibiting] the development of normal activity in the child.

[But] the connection between certain psychic impulses and physical functions is still something else as well. Psychoanalysis was able to show compellingly that certain psychic tendencies could be expressed also physically. Clinical experiences with hysterical and organ-neurotic symptoms offer sufficient evidence for this fact. Headaches as the expression of anger, vomiting as the expression of loathing and repugnance, diarrhoea as the expression of fear are ever repeated signs, alongside which a vast number of others can be placed. We can presuppose the same connection with experiences in the erogenous zones. If the child develops a certain behavior on the grounds of the attitude of the outside world, such as keeping things and refusing to give things up, this behavior will very easily be expressed in the intestinal function. All the more so, the greater the role of this function in early childhood. But also in adults the general tendency to hold back things, to collect and to save, can be expressed in the physical function.

But the conclusion that pleasure in withholding the faeces is the "reason" for pleasure in saving would be just as wrong as, say, the conclusion that headaches are the reason for anger. [In both cases] a definite psychic tendency exists as the expression of a definite attitude to the outside world and the physical sign is *one* form of the expression of this psychic attitude, but not the reason for it. We find the same to be true in regard to dreams. If a parsimonious person dreams that he hoards faeces, Freud would be inclined to interpret this dream in the sense of his theory, so that for the unconscious the said faeces means money which he saves the money because he "actually" wants to save its symbolic equivalent, faeces. But the general principle of the interpretation of dreams, as Freud propounded it, permits of another interpretation in the sense of our conception. We find that dreams readily and frequently employ physical symbols for the expression of more general psychic experiences. This means only that dreams translate psychic experiences into their symbol language, but is no proof that the physical experience is the reason for the psychic.

The conception suggested here leads to a criticism of type forming as in the idea of anal or oral characters. Certainly it is arbitrary from what point of view a type is formed. The forming of a type depends upon what, in the whole phenomenon, is at the time the focal point of interest, or what the main interest is from the point of view of which the various phenomena are to be compared. Psychological types, like those of introversion and extraversion, can be formed if above all the interest lies in differentiating people by their relations to the outside world or to themselves. Types like those of hysterical or compulsion neurosis characters can be formed if above all the interest lies in emphasizing differences in regard to certain behavior as most purely expressed in certain neurotic symptoms. Types like those of domineering, greedy or sado-masochistic characters can be formed if the interest lies in the particular behavior of conduct anchored in the character structure of the personality.

It is expected of all type forming that it be adequate to the scientific interest by which it is determined. This is not the case in the forming of types like the anal and oral character. The guiding point of view in these types is a genetic one. The type is supposed to differentiate people according to what the root of their character structure is. If it is assumed that the condition for the uniformity of the "anal" character syndrome is not the uniformity of the erogenous zones, but the uniformity of a definite outside world constellation to which the individual reacts in the sense of developing those character traits, then it follows that a genetic type forming must not be centered around the erogenous zones but around the typical constellation that conditions the definite character structures. As far as our interest lies in character beyond certain individual differences, such constellations are social ones.

We find that what Freud describes as anal character is actually, in its most pronounced form, the average character of the European lower middle-classes. Hence, from the genetic point of view, a forming a type like that of the lower middle-class character seems to us a possible, genetically orientated [option] and, in any case, a scientifically more correct one than that of the "anal" character. If the interest lies in a character structure that forms a still broader framework than that of the lower middle-classes, types like the "middle-class character" will be encountered.

4. The outcome of the revised psychoanalytic theory: the socially formed character

a) The socially typical character representing the socially moulded psychic structure of the individual

Until now we have spoken essentially about impulses and character syndromes as they are found in individuals and have tried to show that these are not to be understood as direct products of the sexual instinct, but as reactions to certain outside-world conditions and—in the broadest sense—as object relations.

Society and the individual are not "opposite" to each other. *Society is nothing but living, concrete individuals, and the individual can live only as a social human being.* His individual life practice is necessarily determined by the life practice of his society or class and, in the last analysis, by the manner of production of his society, that is, how this society produces, how it is organized to satisfy the needs of its members. The differences in the manner of production and life of various societies or classes lead to the development of different character structures typical of the particular society. Various societies differ from each other not only in differences in manner of production and social and political organization but also in that their people exhibit a typical character structure despite all individual differences. We shall call this the *"socially typical character"*.

Socially typical character is a category that is necessarily less specific than individual character. In describing the character of an individual we are dealing with the totality of this character's many traits which, in their special configuration, go to make up this very character. Just as in all type forming, in the socially typical character only certain fundamental traits are distinguished and these are such as in their dynamic nature and their weight, are of decisive importance for all individuals of this society. The fruitfulness of this category is proved in the fact that, despite the generality of the type, it is still specific to the society in question and stands out from the socially typical character of other societies; further, that analysis also traces back the individual's character with all his individual traits to the elements of the socially typical character and that an understanding of socially typical character is essential to a full understanding of individual character. In class societies the members of the various classes exhibit a common socially typical character that, while holding true for all them, is augmented by certain traits holding true only for the particular class in a configuration typical of this class.

Before going any further into the problem of the socially typical character it is necessary to recall again the fundamental conception of character such as psychoanalysis has propounded it and such as holds true also for the modification of the Freudian libido theory suggested above. Character is not the sum of a person's typical, manifest attitudes and behavior, but the structure of those impulses, fears and attitudes which, for the most part unconsciously, determine the person's typical, manifest behavior. It is especially important here to understand the dynamic quality of character: in it forces are at work which are bound and canalized in the character trait [in a quite specific way]. Character is the form in which a large portion of human energy finds its expression, the tool of the individual, so to speak, loaded with impulse energy with which he carries out his needs under the given life conditions and protects himself against dangers.

b) The function of the socially typical character

The socially typical character varies in its make-up just as does the manner of production and life of various social formations and the classes within them. However, its make-up is always particularly related to the duties a certain individual must perform—in a narrow sense his economic occupation, in a broader sense his social conduct—and to the prohibitions he must respect, especially the necessity of subordinating himself to a ruling class. As far as the performing of certain duties is concerned, the [real] necessity to satisfy needs in a certain way, to act in a certain way in order to avert starvation, is certainly the decisive motive for the particular conduct of an individual. But the greater the intensity of work necessary in a certain society, the more complicated the duties the individual must perform; at the same time, the more alien these duties are to the human needs of the individual, the more the rational cognizance of the necessity for exacted behavior proves an insufficient motive. And for two reasons: The first reason is that intensive and differentiated accomplishment requires a degree of energy and interest which mere force or mere cognizance of the necessity for certain behavior does not supply. [Activities] like building, extensive agriculture or the work of an unqualified factory worker can, of course, be performed on the grounds of pure necessity, but qualified activities require "free will."

The individual must want to do the thing he does or to conduct himself the way he does; the externally necessary must become internally desirable. Here we come to the other reason: In a social order in which the individual is politically free, a degree of subjective satisfaction is required in order that he function satisfactorily and without friction. Of course, a certain [activity] or way of life could bring with it this satisfaction if it conformed to the human needs of the individual, if it were an expression of his individuality. But if the exacted occupation or manner of conduct is alien to him, externally imposed, then this satisfaction must come by way of developing a character structure on the basis of which the socially necessary becomes something satisfying to the individual, something he strives for and accomplishes.

The members of a tribe that lives by war and plunder must develop pleasure in fighting, plundering and personal glory. The members of a tribe that carries on intensive agriculture on a co-operative basis must develop a certain devotion to work and a certain degree of friendliness and readiness to help towards one's fellows. The middle-class person must develop a certain degree of aggressiveness in his character structure, a certain intensification of the impulse to earn a livelihood, to work, to compete with others and to want to outdo them; he must repress his own demands for joy and satisfaction for the benefit of the need to fulfill his duty. But through having developed a character structure in which such impulses and attitudes are present, the practice of exacted conduct such as duty-fulfillment, work, competition, etc. becomes somewhat satisfying for him.

To be sure, to satisfy the "psychic existence minimum", i.e. the minimal necessary degree of subjective satisfaction [compatible with] for the functioning of the individual without friction, additional means are required. Such additional satisfactions can for the most part be supplied by ideologies and require no noteworthy material expenditure. In the character structure where the sadistic and masochistic impulses are strongly developed, it is the corresponding arrangements that effect such fantasy satisfactions. The satisfying of these impulses is especially important where the material needs of the person are not sufficiently satisfied, and especially where the material situation is unsatisfying they are produced in considerable quantity. The "circenses" of ancient Rome are the classical example of sadistic fantasy satisfaction. The same is true of narcissistic attitudes. If the person's self-reliance which takes pride in accomplishment and personality is weakened, then this weakening is compensated for by fantasies along the following lines: one's nation or race is the most pre-eminent and best among all peoples and the simple fact of belonging to this group raises the individual above people of all other groups.

The socially typical character, along with impulses and expectations representing an intensification of the necessary and permitted, contains also traits that are an intensification of the forbidden. Also this side of the socially typical character is of great importance for the function of society. The individual, in his social existence, must give up the satisfying of certain impulses for the general good. But beyond that he must give up, in many societies, the satisfying of needs which are not directly connected with his social existence [as such] but with the structure of a certain society.

Middle-class society has made a certain degree of sexual repression and the denial altogether of the demand for happiness necessary; moreover, it has added to this, especially for the broad masses, limitations in satisfaction and enjoyment of material things (even though at the same time [instilling] a taste for this enjoyment) which places these masses in harsh contrast to the wealthy classes. Were these demands vital to the individual and if they had, so to speak, to yield to force each time, then the consequences would be, in the first place, that in many cases the individual would insist upon carrying out his demands in spite of threatening prohibitions; and secondly that even where they are consciously repressed, a resentment and hostility would develop [in the individual] towards those people that compel him to repression. The result would be, seen from the standpoint of society, highly unsatisfactory. The social necessity of an automatic impulse denial, without a development that would lead to strong resentment, demands that the impulses denied satisfaction—whether physiological like sexuality or psychic of some kind—be repressed, that is, they must appear no more as needs in the conscious or in quantitatively lesser degree. The external prohibition becomes an internal one, a demand of the conscience or, as Freud named it in its dynamic aspect, of the "Super-Ego" which, for its part, is the internalization of the authorities ruling a society. (Compare E. Fromm, 1936a.)

The socially typical character is determined by the manner of production and life of a society. But its formation is additionally influenced by a number of other factors, or intensified by certain traits of special social significance. The factors we are dealing with can be described generally as ideological influences. Religion was the strongest instrument of such an influence on character structure; today it has been largely replaced by certain political ideologies. The social function of Protestantism and its sects was considerably responsible for the intensification of those character traits which were already developing from the changed manner of production. But it is more than just a question of the intensification of certain traits.

Religion represents a system that contributes towards integrating character traits developed from the social way of life—that is, not for the purpose of intensifying certain traits but also of producing others which are not merely reflexes of social life but requisites to the formation of the whole character. But at the same time it creates fantasy satisfactions, which are necessary for the person with his definite socially typical character. Protestantism and especially the Protestant sects have begotten fear by their teachings; but at the same time, by stressing duty and what [Max] Weber calls "innerworldly asceticism" showed the way to a relative liberation of this fear; in this way it influences the socially typical character of middle-class society in the direction fundamentally given by the manner of production and life in middle-class society.

Between the economic structure of a society and the socially typical character there exists a certain labile equilibrium. The character is developed in reaction to the given manner of production and it develops psychic needs which, seen from the standpoint of the individual, can be relatively satisfied on a particular level of the manner of production, and which, seen from the standpoint of society, supply the necessary psychic energy for the carrying out of the individual's duties. As long as the circumstance of this labile equilibrium exists, the character tends to strengthen inwardly the existing social relations, especially the class relations. It is, so to speak, the cement that holds the given social structure together. It supplies the impulses that drives the people to do what is bidden, to avoid what is forbidden and to find a certain degree of satisfaction in conforming to existing relations.

But this labile equilibrium is constantly disturbed. As society develops new manner of behavior are demanded which no longer correspond to the formed psychic structure. On the other hand, needs that are anchored in the traditional character structure are no longer satisfied. The capitalist of the trust era, if he wants to be successful, requires other psychic impulses than the businessman of earlier capitalistic stages. For instance, to him the trait to save would be an obstacle rather than help.

An especially good example for this is seen in the relation in dictatorial states. The decline of economic conditions in the lower middle-classes, the structural unemployment brought about by the crisis could no longer satisfy the middle-class character imbedded in needs for economic independence, saving, work and also partly in a growing pleasure in material things. This dissatisfaction of the needs imbedded in the traditional character structure led to the people as a whole becoming more and more dissatisfied with existing conditions so that the needs anchored in the character changed from an element of holding together to one of dissolution and threatening the existing society. Cement, as it were, became dynamite.

The conflict between economic conditions and the given character structure can be removed, schematically speaking, in one of two ways. First, by changing the economic conditions in such a way that the needs which grow out of the existing character structure can be satisfied. The other possibility is when, on grounds of class relations in a certain society, the economic change necessary for the first solution is not acceptable: Then an attempt [must be] made to evolve a character structure whose needs can be satisfied under the given economic conditions. In dictatorial states the attempt is being made to reshape the people inwardly in this sense. An attempt is being made, with every means of propaganda and influence, to create a character with needs for subordination, self-sacrifice, hero worship instead of the traditional middle-class character with needs for personal success, work and happiness.

Nevertheless, it is unavoidable that the ideological influences have but a limited effect on the forming of the character's structure. This is derived, to such a great extent, from the actual life relations of people that the enduring success of an ideology conflicting with these relations is doubtful. Human solidarity, such as develops under the circumstance of numerous workers laboring together on great projects; an certain intellectual level, such as the activities of a qualified worker inculcates; a feeling for individuality, such as comes about in a manner of production in which the individual must accomplish quite complicated feats—are not easy to destroy with ideological influences of an opposing nature.

Let us sum up in short the conception of socially typical character here presented. Human energies appear in social life not in some general form, but are, so to speak, guided into those channels that make them useful to the functioning of a certain society. Character seen from this point of view is the definite form in which psychic energy appears as a productive force in the social process. Or, expressed differently, the socially typical character is a part of the whole social machinery without which it would not function, or not sufficiently.

5. Analytic social psychology compared with other approaches

Social psychology must describe the socially typical character, analyse it on the strength of fundamental unconscious impulses, fears and attitudes present in it, it must show to what extent the socially typical character is a product of the manner of life and production in a society and the ideological influences on the individual that takes place in it, and finally it must show how psychic energies, expressed and formed in character traits enter into the social process as productive forces.

Only the concrete analysis of socially typical characters, which cannot be attempted within the framework of this paper, can prove whether the conceptions here presented are substantiated, no less in regard to whether it succeeds in deriving the socially typical character from the manner of production and life in a society, than in regard to whether the knowledge of the socially typical character sharpens insight into social dynamics.

The theory of a socially typical character here presented deals with a theme which, since Lazarus and Steintal's "Völkerpsychologie", again and again has been dealt with from the most varying points of view, for various motives and with various methods. We want to touch upon short three treatments which are especially closely related to our problem: a) The German-English discussion on the "spirit" of society, b) the theory of historical materialism, and c) the American perceptions of "pattern" and "habits" as stamping the personality of a particular society.

a) Approaches to exploring the "spirit" of a society

The problem of the "spirit" of society was argued on the example of the "middle-class" spirit.[13] Sombart calls the "spirit" of an economy "the totality of psychic traits which are in play in social production. All expressions of the intellect, all the character traits that come forth in productive striving, equally thought, likewise too set aims, all judgments of value, all fundamental propositions by which the behavior of the productive man is determined and regulated." (W. Sombart, 1923, p. 2.)

Max Weber saw the "spirit" of capitalism in its connection with Protestantism and Protestant sects. He tries to show that Protestantism has produced in middle-class people just those traits that are of decisive significance for his behavior as a productive person in capitalism. The theory of pre-determination and the theory that man cannot influence God by doing good works created in middle-class people, according to Weber, the need to

13 Compare especially: W. Sombart, 1923; M. Weber, 1920; R. H. Tawney, 1927; L. J. Brentano, 1916; E. Troeltsch, 1919; L. Kraus, 1930.

prove to himself by [getting on] in his professional activity, by success in his economic occupation, that God has blessed him. This constant seeking after a visible sign of God's blessing has led to an "inner-worldly asceticism" that is, becoming reconciled with or receiving a sign of blessing from God by unceasing toil, fulfillment of one's duties and striving for success. Despite all the justified objections raised against Weber during the discussion, the fact remains that he saw correctly certain decisive traits of the middle-class person in which a connection between his professional activity and the Protestant religion exists. Even such a firm critic of Weber's as Kraus, admits that Weber is right when he says, "that the appraisal of duty fulfillment within worldly occupations as the highest content moral exemplification could assume, was unknown to the old church as well as the church of the Middle Ages." (L. Kraus, 1930, p. 245.)

Our chief objection to Weber's theory is that he sees the relation turned upside down and this in two ways. For one thing, Weber traces back the peculiarities of the middle-class person to the special content of Protestantism; he explains the middle-class person by his religious ideas and not the ideas by a person who is stamped by a definite form of economics. And for another Weber sees the relations of the people themselves turned upside down. He believes that the ideas a person has and especially the religious ideas determine his conduct, and does not see that the ideas are themselves an expression of impulses and fears for the most part unconscious that are present in people, that is, of his character structure, taken in the dynamic sense. Religious ideologies could only come about on a definitely socially typical characterological basis or be effective on the basis of the socially typical character. This is the immediate foundation for the conscious content but it is itself determined by the manner of production and life of the society. Religion, as we have tried to indicate above, has the role of intensifying and integrating the character structure determined by the particular kind of economics.

Weber refuses any attempt at understanding middle-class character in the sense of a psychological theory. Sombart makes this attempt but in a most superficial way. A characteristic example of this are the false and superficial psychological categories with which he works. As for instance, when he says of the pre-capitalist person: "That is the natural person. The person as God created him. . . . therefore, to discover his economic disposition is not difficult: it arises out of human nature of its own accord." (W. Sombart, 1923, p. 11.) [Or when he states:] "As a matter of fact the psychic structure of the modern entrepreneur as well as all modern people infected with his spirit, seems to me best understood if one steps into the child's world of imagination and values and brings to consciousness the fact that in the entrepreneurs who appear to us larger than life-size, and [indeed] in all really modern people the driving forces of their dealings are the same as in the child. These people's final evaluations mean a tremendous reduction of all psychic processes to their simplest elements, they represent a complete simplification of psychic experiences, they are a kind of regression to the simple conditions in the child's soul. I [will even back up this view.] The child has four elementary complexes of values, four 'ideals' rule his life: 1. the [sensory dimension]; 2. quick motion; 3. the new; 4. the sense of power. These—and if we examine them closely, only these—ideals of the child are behind all specific modern notions of value." (W. Sombart, 1923, pp. 221f.)

What is the opposing theoretical position suggested here? We conceive what is understood as the "spirit" of a society or a human type to be a conscious expression of the socially typical character structure and we try to analyse and examine the character structure of the middle-class person, above all also its unconscious elements, and the extent to which this character structure is an expression of the people's manner of life, specific for capitalist production. Such an analysis would proceed from the basic relation of people to other people created by capitalist production—his monadic isolation, the fear that arises from the absolute instability of the economic situation, his psychic isolation and the constantly produced conscious, and still more unconscious, hostility towards other people [induced] by competition. It would examine to what extent this fundamental structure leads to a deep need for justification which, for its part, is satisfied by duty fulfillment and success. It would have to show how the capitalistic manner of economics changes all things, people as well, into commodities towards which only an indirect, estranged relation exists, and to what extent the possibility of satisfying all desires by means of money cripples the inner activity of people and the capacity for expression, and to what extent only the capacity to earn money is developed. The "spirit" of capitalism is not a [fixed] point by which we can explain people; the character structure of the middle-class person must be analysed; the spirit must be understood in its rootedness in the character structure and this itself by virtue of the manner of production and life of the people.

The decisive basic criticism of theories, like Sombart's, that explain historical phenomena by an idea prevalent in a particular epoch or by a certain spirit, was made in Marx's criticism of Proudhon. "Let us assume for the moment with Mr. Proudhon that actual history is chronologically the historical succession in which the ideas, the categories, the principles manifested themselves. Each principle had its century in which it was disclosed. The dictatorial principle had for instance, the 11th century, just as the principle of individualism had the 18th. Logically, the century belongs to the principle, not the principle to the century. In other words: the principle makes history, not history the principle. If, to rescue the principles and history, one asks: why these principles manifested themselves particularly in the 11th and 18th centuries and not in some other centuries, then one finds oneself necessarily forced to examine in detail: What were the people of the 11th and 18th centuries, what were their needs at the different times, their forces of production, their manner of production, the raw materials of their production, what, finally, were the relations of person to person that took place by reason of all these conditions of existence? To fathom all these questions, isn't this, to penetrate the actual profane history of the people as they were, the author and producer of their own drama? But the instant the people are presented as the authors and producers of their own history then one has arrived back again through a detour to the actual starting point because the eternal principles with which one started have been dropped." (K. Marx, *Das Elend der Philosophie*, 1971, p. 503.)

b) The theory of historical materialism

The Marx-Engels theory did not assume, as has been widely represented in many interpretations of historical materialism, that the decisive principle of explanation of history is the human drive to earn a living. The economic consideration was not a subjective psychological motive for them, but the objective condition of human life activity and of social development. Marx and Engels understood the individual and his consciousness by his social being. "People are the makers of their imagination, ideas, etc., but the actual, effective people are determined by a particular development of their forces of production and by the corresponding traffic with these forces up to its widest formations." (K. Marx, *Die Deutsche Ideologie*, MEGA I, 5, p. 15.) They noted the dependence of "culture", of the ideological super-structure upon the economic sub-structure, saw in the spiritual "material things transformed in the human-mind." These material things were, however, not their physical organization, but their material life process, whose psychic motor is the tendency to satisfy human needs. Historical materialism has shown that the human being and his thoughts are products of their manner of production and that these are "a certain kind of activity of these individuals, a certain way of expressing their life, a certain manner of life of these people." (K. Marx, *Die Deutsche Ideologie*, MEGA I, 5, p. 15.)

They have not dealt with the problem of how material things, in concrete detail, "are transformed in the human mind", which in concrete detail is the mediator between super-structure and sub-structure. Engels distinctly stresses this in a letter to Mehring (of July 14th, 1893, quoted from H. Duncker, 1930): "Namely all of us have primarily laid, and have had to lay, the main stress on deriving of the political, legal and other ideological conceptions, and the conduct introduced by these conceptions, from the economic facts. In so doing we have neglected the formal aspect over the contents: the ways and means by which these conceptions come about."

This is the point where an analytical social psychology has its place within the theory of historical materialism. It can show in detail that the people's manner of production and life creates quite a definite character structure and that the consciousness of people, in so far as it is not directly a rational reflex thrown up by social practice, is determined by the special form of people's drives, fears and expectations, especially the unconscious ones. Social psychological theory is all the more important the more it has to do with people's irrational manner of conduct—which, however, despite its irrationality, is not to be explained by "madness", but by the character structure formed in the social process.

The modification of the Freudian theory suggested in this work seems to us in some respects to stand closer to the theory of historical materialism than to the Freudian libido theory. This shares with Marx's and Engels' points of view a fundamental skepticism towards the consciousness of people; also a dialectical interpretation of psychic processes. The partly direct tracing back of spiritual and psychic phenomena to immediate physiological sources conforms, however, to a mechanistic materialistic philosophy that was surmounted in dialectical materialism. Certainly, the physical organization of the person and his physiological needs enter as a decisive factor into his whole life practice. The theory here suggested stands closer to the viewpoints of historical materialism than the Freudian ones, insofar as the psychic structure of man is regarded as the product of his activity and his manner of life and not as the reflex thrown up by his physical organization. This life practice determines the socially typical character, which is one of the most important mediators between super—and sub-structure and the particular form in which psychic energy enters into the social process as productive force.[14]

c) The concept of "habits" in American social psychology

In American social psychological literature the most widespread conception is to regard traits as they appear typically in the individual of a society as "habits," stamped directly by the customs, technologies, the "patterns" of a society. The category

14 [Compare for the relation to the theory of historical materialism our more detailed presentation in E. Fromm, 1932a, further W. Reich, 1929, and R. Osborn, 1937.]

that is the center of this conception is "behavior." These conceptions, as they have developed especially in the struggle against instinct theories indicate an advance over Sombart and Weber insofar as they invest the social factors with a greater role than the others do (even though [getting bogged down in the environmental] theory) and represent a tilt at the psychological theories that explain society by human drives. They are lacking, however, in two directions. They treat "habits" of people mechanistically as a sum of single traits and do not see the structuredness of behavior as a whole, that is the fact that all single traits of people are intertwined in quite a definite way and mutually determine each other. In this regard the picture drawn by Weber and Sombart, despite all its other shortcomings, was far superior.

The other flaw in the theory centered around "behavior" is that behavior is accepted as the last unit and the question is not asked, what are the unconscious impulses, fears and attitudes that determine particular behavior, in other words, what is the character structure out of which particular behavior grows? Certainly, there are a great number of socially typical manners of behavior that essentially are nothing but the taking over of socially given "patterns". Manners of behavior of this kind would be, let us say, customs like the manner of greeting, eating or many others of a similar nature. But as far as—and all the more when—we are dealing with forms of behavior that are relevant to the functioning of society as well as also to the personality of the individual, a full understanding demands the analysis of personality structure. Only in connection with the knowledge of character structure can it be understood why the socially given "pattern" of the people of this society can be accepted and practised with great intensity.

Certain behavior, although seeming just like some other under rough external observation, will differ in people as well in regard to its minute details—as in regard to the emotional depth of its anchorage—if the character structure is different. A trait like the tendency to acquisitiveness is usually regarded in the American conception here cited as a social technique or custom which is given the individual by society and used by him. Social psychological analysis shows, however, that acquisitiveness in its specific peculiarity and in the intensity it assumes as a tendency in the middle-class person, can only be understood on the basis of his character structure. Let us take a socially typical character quite different from the middle-class one, like the Pueblo Indian or the pre-capitalistic European individual—then the quantity and quality of acquisitiveness, as far as it can be found at all as an essential trait, is altogether different. Were acquisitiveness to be introduced as a "pattern" in a society with a socially typical character of quite another nature, it could either not be practised at all by the people or only with negligible energy. Only if on grounds of changes in the social relation the whole socially typical character in this society is changed, and in the sense that acquisitiveness is made a need supplied and carried from within, could this habit become effective in the sense it is in modern people. A number of tribes still behind in capitalistic development are a living example for this.[15]

The same holds true not only for "patterns" of certain manners of behavior but also for all ideologies. A certain ideology, like that of duty fulfillment or success as the decisive content and goal of life, becomes effective only on the basis of a quite definite character structure. Certainly, it also contributes towards

15 [Compare with the beautiful examples of the lack of acquisitiveness that are given in Bertram Wolf's book on the Mexican Indian, 1937.]

forming the character structure, as we have seen above, but this is determined in its decisive elements by the manner of life in the society. The same ideology that is impressive to and effective in the middle-class character would have meant nothing but words to the character of the pre-capitalistic person. The effectiveness of an ideology does not depend upon a rational rightness or comprehension but upon certain emotional presuppositions as they are given with the character structure.

Our conception is that typical forms of behavior by people and their readiness to accept certain ideologies cannot essentially be regarded directly as reflexes thrown up by, or taking over of, social "patterns"; rather then are supplied and carried by a character structure that is, for its part, the product of the specific life practice and in the sense presented above, the adjustment of the person within the given natural and social conditions with the goal of satisfying his physiological and historically created needs.[16]

16 [An American conception that is, to be sure, centered around the idea of "habits," but on the other hand also takes into account psychic impulses and desires is John Dewey's theory. He designates as the problem of social psychology "not how either individual or collective mind forms social groups and customs, but how different customs, established interacting arrangements, form and nurture different minds." (J. Dewey, 1922, p. 63.) Dewey takes a certain middle position between MacDougall's theory and a behavioristic orientation. Although we agree in many details with his formulations—as also the one quoted—his theory seems to us unsatisfactory in so far as he has not seen the necessity for an analysis of character structure and especially its unconscious portions.]

II. PSYCHIC NEEDS AND SOCIETY (LECTURE 1956)

What matters for the understanding of man's nature are the specific conditions of human existence. Man is an animal and he is not an animal. Man is within nature and he transcends nature. Man is, if you please, a freak of nature. He is the only life being aware of itself. And this particular situation of being within nature and transcending it, of having self-awareness, and having a minimum of instinctual developments, creates in man a peculiar situation which is the human situation. The animal essentially is guided in his life and action by his instincts. The animal's life is lived by the equipment and endowment nature has given it. Man has very little of that.

Man has to live his own life and is from the day of his birth confronted with a question to which he has to answer. The question arising from the dichotomies of human existence, the special conditions of human existence. I cannot go too far into this but nevertheless I want to mention it briefly.

(1) Man *has to be related to others*. If man is not related he is insane. And in fact this is the only valid definition of insanity, the person who is absolutely unrelated, the person—as Ibsen

put it in *Peer Gynt*—is himself and nothing but himself. Man inasmuch as he is not insane has to be related but he can relate himself in several ways. Just to give two ways: he can relate himself in a symbiotic way, namely either by submitting to somebody or by having power over somebody, but this other person being necessary for him to live at all. On the other hand, he can relate himself by love, by which I mean to be one with another person under the condition of separateness, under the condition of integrity of the two. Whether he is related in one way or the other that makes the differentia between health and not health. But he has to be related in some way if he is to be sane at all. You might say just as man can eat many kinds of food, some good for him and some bad for him, but if he wouldn't eat at all he would die. And death, in the physiological realm is the same as insanity is in the mental realm.

(2) The second need of man again based on the conditions of human existence is he *has to be rooted somewhere.* We all come from mother's womb. We all come from nature. What does it mean that we are born? Actually we overestimate the act of birth tremendously, the physiological act of birth, because the baby after his birth in many ways is much more like the fetus than the grown-up person is like the baby. The only difference is, he is now bodily, physiologically outside of mother; he is nourished by his own system; and he has to breathe. Breathing is the first activity necessary if the separation from mother is to take place. But for quite a long time the baby remains just the same, completely dependent on mother much longer than any animal, and then there is a slow process of development.

Birth is an act which continues through life, namely emerging from the ties of mother and nature into a person of one's own. The tragedy of life is that most of us die before we are fully born. But you can almost characterize any person by pointing to the point where he stopped to be born. The psychotic person is stopped in his birth already in the womb because his longing is to return to the womb, to return to death, to return to pre-consciousness and pre-individuality. The receptive person who lives a life always expecting somebody to nourish him, to give him something, to be kind to him, is stopped at birth and at mother's breast, and so on and so on.

There is a continuous process, a process in which we cut down ties to the past, ties to the mother, and emerge into a new situation which we can manage only by our own activities. That is why breathing is so important, not only physiologically but psychologically and symbolically. Just as the act of separation from mother at the time of birth is possible only by the first act of activity, namely breathing, any separation, any act of being born, is psychologically possible only by assuming a new activity of our own.

Actually I believe we can observe in any person two tendencies: a wish to return and a wish to be born. Or you can put it differently: a fear to emerge from that which is certain, from the ties of the past, and at the same time a wish to remove one's self from the presence of this certainty and the past into a new situation, into a new activity. I believe that what Freud described as the death instinct and life instinct may be more accurately described by the two tendencies; namely, the one for aggression and the one for birth.

Every act of birth, every step into the new, is uncertain and is something we fear. You might say it requires faith. Certain is only the past and we might say the only certain thing is death. In any act of birth, in any progress, in any evolution, in any emergence, there is uncertainty, but there is at the same time the tendency in human nature to want to emerge from the past because the past appears at a certain point as a chain. Neurosis however can be defined, and psychosis too, as an inability to be born beyond a certain point. Incidentally what we call neurosis and psychosis I think to a large extent is culturally determined. That is to say, we call normal anyone who is as crazy as the average, or who is as little born or as little developed as the average is.

(3) Now another need is our *need to transcend*. We are born as creatures and yet we cannot stand the idea of being like dice thrown out of a cup. We want to transcend our creatureliness, our creature nature, and we can do it in two ways. We can create life. Women can do it anyway by nature. Men can't do it that way so they do it by ideas or all sorts of things. We can transcend life by creation. But creation is difficult in many ways and if we cannot transcend life by creation, we can transcend life by destruction. Destroying life is just as much transcending it as creating it. Destructiveness is so to speak a secondary potentiality in man. If we cannot cope with life by creating or if we cannot transcend life by creating, we try to transcend it by destroying, and in the act of destruction we make ourselves superior to life.

(4) Another need is our *need for identity*. We have to be able to say "I". If we can't say "I" we are crazy, again. But we can say "I" in many ways. In the primitive tribe you might find the concept of I as being expressed by the we. I is we. There is no sense of individuality outside of the belonging to the tribe. Now we live not in a primitive tribe today. We live in a period in which all the original, organic ties of family, of tribe and of blood have broken down to a tremendous extent. Man today is confronted with the possibility of developing the sense of "I" but that means he has developed his own creativity, his own productivity, he has to be he, he has to sense himself, experience himself, as a center and subject of his own action. If he can't do that, there is only one other solution and that is conformity.

He must conform to the rest and he feels he is "I" as long as he is no different from his neighbor. If he gets three feet away he is already frightened because then the problem of his identity, "who am I," really starts being sensed by him. As long as he conforms absolutely he has no need to ask, "Who am I," because obviously "I am as the rest of us."

(5) And eventually there is a *need for some frame of orientation and devotion*. We have to have some picture of life, this picture of the world, as we have to have a spatial picture in order to be able to walk. This can be rational, it can be irrational. From this concept you start out with the real conditions of human existence. You start out with an analysis of what is man, what is his nature, what are the specific conditions of his existence, and then you try to find out what are the basic needs and passions which follow from this condition, from his existence, and in what way can he answer these needs. I am trying to say he can answer them in different ways and these ways make the difference between mental health and mental illness.

Now this is actually the difference between a physiological concept, in which you take the isolated individual with the chemical processes in him as creating certain tensions which have to be reduced and man relating to each other as mutual means to the purpose of this satisfaction, as against a biological concept and an existentialist concept. In the latter you do not start out primarily with a model of man as being a machine with certain tensions which need reduction, but you start out with the very conditions of man's existence, and the needs arising from it and man's relatedness to other men and to the world outside of him, as the *primary datum* given from which then you can understand and explain certain passions, certain fears, and certain necessities.

Another point of a more sociological nature has immediate

relevance to the whole topic I am talking about. Freud thought always of society, as it was quite characteristic for the nineteenth century as society per se. Of course, he knew there were different societies but essentially Freud was thinking of society as a repressive agent and societies varied for him only in terms of the degree of the repression. Primitive society, according to him, which is quite wrong objectively, didn't repress at all and modern society repressed a great deal, and society varied to the degree to which they repressed the innate destructiveness and egocentricity of man.

What Freud did not see, and what was not in the kind of intellectual atmosphere he personally was living in although there were others who saw such things, was that there is no such thing as society per se. There are very different societies with different structures and with different roles that men and women have in them. It is not just a matter of quantity of repression more or less but a difference of quality of an entirely different structure.

From the standpoint of society, an individual has to fulfill certain roles which fit into the structure of society. In the nineteenth century people had to be economical and thrifty and not to waste money because it was a society in which it was important to accumulate capital. In the twentieth century, people have to spend a lot and consume a lot because it is an economy which is based on ever increasing production. Now, in a society of warriors, you have to be an individualist and to defy death and to be proud in fame. In a society of an agricultural tribe which has a method of production and of cooperation, you have to act quite differently.

The point is that people don't choose these roles. They don't decide consciously "I want to be this and I want to be that." Actually this is a matter of character. Thriftiness, or the pleasure in consuming, or the pleasure in glory and in war, or the pleasure in peaceful cooperations—all these are character traits. The aim of society, if it wants to survive in its particular structure, is that everybody wants to do what he has to do. The social role assigned to him and the behavior assigned to him is not a matter of his decision every time but is a matter of his character. He assumes a character which guarantees, so to speak, that most people without questioning will act in the way they need to act for the existence and survival of this society.

In the middle ages punctuality was unknown. In Mexico this is still somewhat the case. Nobody would particularly worry whether it is eight o'clock or eight thirty. In fact, the clock that struck the half hour happened for the first time in the sixteenth century. Why? Because to the work he was doing it was of no importance to be five minutes or a half hour early or late. It is obvious that in our modern industrial organization punctuality is terribly important. You just couldn't function without a sense of time and without a sense of orderliness. Punctuality and orderliness have become character traits. You don't decide to be punctual or orderly, but you are by character.

As long as the economical and social conditions which existed in the past continues to exist, then there is no problem. The traditional character trait is produced by the parental character, by ideas, by books, by schools, and so on, fit with the necessity of society. When you have considerable changes in society, when you need new human attitudes because society requires it, then you have very often the profound conflict that your traditional social character is not in line anymore with the more recent requirement of society. We are today in such a situation. Our traditional character is one still of individuality and our present day social necessities as they are rooted in our social life are quite different.

Then you very often get sudden changes which lead to a

kind of anarchy, to a kind of emptiness, to a kind of vacuum, because there is not yet sufficient integration, or sufficient tradition, to create that new type of social character which is required. In many centuries, the process of change is so slow that the two lines, namely that of social and economic development on the one hand and character development on the other, can adjust to each other. Then you have no violent periods of chaos. Sometimes it is very great like today and you have real problems.

But this is looking at man from the standpoint of society, from the needs of a given society and its own survival. Now I don't mean to say society thinks or society does anything, but a social system has its own logic, its own dynamisms and it requires a certain kind of behavior and feeling in order to function. And if one looks at man from the standpoint of does he feel the need of society, as many people do, then all that matters is that his behavior and his character fit into the necessities of society.

I believe this is only one side of the question. Man is not only a member of society. Man is a member of the human race. Man has necessities of his own which exist quite independently from any other society. It is true that man has to live in such a way that he will fill the demands of society, but it is also true that society has to be constructed and structuralized in such a way that it will fill the needs of man. The needs of man are the needs which very briefly I tried to sketch before. If you have a society like the Stalinist or Nazi society in which man loses the sense of love and human solidarity, you do something to man which is against his necessities as man; that is to say, man as a member of the human race. You might define a good society as a society which approaches most meeting the needs of humanity, the needs of man, and a bad society as society in which the gap between human needs and social needs is great. I think there is a point in which man either becomes pathological and breaks down, and so society breaks down, or in such a society he tries to change the society in such a way as to make it more human. The conflict however always exist.

The conflict between the historical need of any given society to make man function and the human needs based in the essence of human existence to make man function, and it is a matter of decision and conscience to anybody what is God's and what is Caesar's, what is society's and what is man's. Any society can be analyzed and can be judged in terms of this conflict and it is up to any individual to see what he owes to conformity and what he owes to sanity. Sometimes conformity can be insanity and I don't mean that just figuratively speaking.

I have tried to indicate a different point of view in terms of man and society as Freud had it. Freud saw society primarily as repressive. I see society as partly repressive and partly creative. Out of society, outside of social life, outside of social contacts, man couldn't develop at all. And society does not only have the function to repress the evil instincts which are in man. Society has also the function, and more so I would say, to develop the human potentialities which are given in the human race.

III. DEALING WITH THE UNCONSCIOUS IN PSYCHOTHERAPEUTIC PRACTICE (3 LECTURES 1959)

1. My understanding of what is being unconscious

If one uses the term, "repression," as it is used usually by Freud and as it is used in analytic literature, one thinks primarily of something which *was* conscious and then was repressed. While in my concept here I refer to that which is not conscious, in equal ways, both to that which had been conscious, and to that which we had never been aware of. Therefore, perhaps it would be better, maybe to word the term, "*dissociation*," rather than "repression," because in the term "dissociation" you have more of a possibility to comprise both: that which has arrived and that which has not arrived in awareness. It has not quite the active pushing back quality. In order to give another example for that kind of dissociations which I had in mind as being that which we are not aware of, take a very simple example: You have seen the face of a person, let us say, who is well known to you; you have known him for many years, and one day you suddenly see the face entirely afresh. Suddenly, you see this face with what you would describe as simply a greater degree of reality. You know the face; you could describe it, you see a quality, you see an essence, which is much more real than anything you have seen before, and actually for a moment you have the feeling, "I have never seen this face before, it is completely new." What has happened? You are aware of something in the reality of this face of which you have not been aware before. The face was always the same, that is to say the man or the woman was always the same; you are always the same, but you had a veil and you didn't see. You were, what one might say, half blind and suddenly your eyes open and you see.

The whole process really of making the unconscious conscious is a process which could be described as seeing, and actually you have in the mythological literature, the symbol of blindness, utter blindness, and then you become a seer. Tyreseus is blind and he's a seer. Oedipus becomes blinds and he becomes eventually a seer. Faust, in Goethe's *Faust*, becomes blind at the very moment where he sees and he says then, an inner radiance came out from him.

This concept of repression in which one speaks of not being aware of that which exists in myself has the premise that *really all is in us*. Or, if you put it differently, that we know everything, except that we don't know what we know. If I assume, I have never before seen you as I see you now, then I must in my way of putting it, assume I really knew you before but I was not aware of what I was knowing. If I had not known you before, if I had been really blind, then I could only speak of a new insight, rather than of a hidden suppressed, unconscious insight which emerged.

Indeed, I believe we really have everything in us, not only in the sense we are all human and that there is nothing human which is alien to us, because, there is nothing human which is not in us, from the child, to the criminal, to the insane person, to the saint, to the average person. But, I would say, we also are aware of all that, but we are not aware; we sense it. This one of the reasons why pointing to reality which, in my way of thinking, means the same—has such a peculiar effect on people. Because the truth touches only upon something which they know, and once this chord is touched they almost cannot help responding.

The lie does not touch upon reality, the lie touches on nothing, and therefore you can say a thousand lies, because you touch nothing: you touched fiction, you touched unreality, but once you touch reality, which means you say the truth, then something in the person tends to respond, because what you say hits upon that which he knows and yet does not know. Naturally I don't mean the process is so simple, that the person does necessarily respond because there can be such defenses against his own responding—that's what we call resistance, that he will not respond. But, nevertheless, I would say this is the hope for the human race, that in fact the truth makes us free, as the new testament says [John 8:32].

In us is a sense of reality—of our inner reality and of the reality outside—to which one can appeal with a true word. If one couldn't do that, then I think the analytic method would really be essentially impossible, except as a method of persuasion. There is a very interesting Jewish Talmudic myth about this which says, that before the child is born, it knows everything, but to be born with this knowledge would be so painful, that out of mercy an angel touches the child and does away with all his knowledge. What I say here corresponds pretty much to this myth. Unconsciously we know everything and yet we don't, because it is indeed very painful to know and at the same time there is nothing more exhilarating which doesn't even exclude pain than to know, than to be in touch with reality.

Another point I should like to stress is the *connection between individual repression and social repression.* It is true that we mostly have to do with social repression and that there are only individual variants, individual deviation, which work above the social repressions, and they make for more or less repression in this or that area.

How does social and individual repression work together? If you take for instance a mother who gets anxious every time the child does something "bad" and then she has a reaction, the child senses this anxiety, and the child becomes highly sensitive to the notion "bad." To take a mother who is obsessional compulsive, and whose fear of badness is a good deal more intense than that of the average person—take the nineteenth century cultures—then indeed this mother may have been thirty percent above the average obsession with good and bad. But, nevertheless, this child will have great difficulties in getting over the anxiety produced by mother's anxiety about good and badness, because of the culture in which it finds itself; nevertheless, this is supported by the whole culture, the culture never denies the basic principle of the mother's influence. And, of courses in general, we must not forget, the mother, the father, the family are not accidental individuals which occur in a culture, they are formed by the society, that is to say, the child in the first few years is rarely in touch with society as such. But it is in touch with its agents, namely the parents whose character is formed itself by society and whose sociological function is to prepare the child characterologically to become that which the society wants.

If the parents are really crazy—and by really crazy I don't mean it in a psychiatric sense, but I mean to be completely different from the culture in which they live—then the child actually has a much better chance to get away, not to be impressed by the influences. In fact, really crazy for better or worse, that doesn't matter. Once a child grows up a little bit more these parents are then really shown up as being outside of the majority, outside of what is considered to be reasonable, normal, and so on.

Let me say a few words more about the concept of unawareness of experience. What really happens when we have an *experience*? Let me give an example: We have a ball and we throw the ball and the ball rolls, and we say: "The ball rolls." What do we actually experience when we say "The ball rolls?" I think we experience only the following: Our mind confirms our knowledge that a round object on a relatively smooth surface, when pushed, rolls. In other words, when we say: "The ball rolls," we make an intellectual statement that really amounts to saying that we can speak. We know this is a ball and we know the law of nature that the ball rolls. But what happens to a little boy of four when the ball rolls? It happens that he really sees the ball rolling. That is an entirely different experience; it is a beautiful experience; it's an experience—you can call it an ecstatic experience—in which the whole body participates in this beautiful thing of seeing a ball rolling. Some of us for instance, have this experience more clearly when we see people playing tennis. Let us assume that we are not interested in who wins, but we just follow the beautiful movement of the ball going forth and back. The simple act of a rolling ball to us usually appears boring after the second time. Why are we bored? Because we feel we know already that the ball rolls. But for the little boy, it is not a matter that he knows it. For the little boy it is a matter of seeing this movement which is a full experience.

Together with some other people I believe that any thought

which is not dissociated already is not only a thought of our brain, but a thought of our *body*. We think with our muscles; we think with everything in our body. If we think not with our body, if our body is not participating in a thought, then it is already a dissociated thought. Then I do know it is true in thoughts about things, about people. If you, for instance, see a little teddy bear with a very smooth, nice surface, and you see it and you say: "Isn't that beautiful," but you don't feel something in your fingers, the impulse to stroke it, I would say your statement: "It is beautiful" wasn't true. It was one of these statements which we make every day a thousand times: "Isn't it nice," "I feel fine,"—but really you have not had the experience, which allegedly is contained in the sentence: "It is beautiful."

Somebody sees a mountain. What is the first question? "What's the name, what's the altitude?" Once he knows these data cerebrally, he files it away. You see a person and ask: "Who are you?"—and you expect first the name, then the age, then the marriage status—in other words, the passport. Actually, this is beautifully expressed in Ibsen's *Peer Gynt*, where Peer Gynt, when he begins to doubt his identity, eventually asks himself: "Who am I?" and, he answers: "My passport." These are the data which are experienced as "I"—and there is where it ends.

In our way of speaking, in our way of saying, "this is me," or "this is I," "a ball rolls," "this is a rose," "this is a mountain," we are already dissociating from the total experience, the affective part, and are already making a statement. It sounds like a full statement, but is actually a dissociated statement because we are not aware of the affective experience which exists and yet which does not come into awareness. There is the point where the unconscious really begins in daily life.

You do not understand any person unless you know that *life is paradoxical*, and therefore that you have to think paradoxically in order to understand it. A few examples will serve the material which I have presented, or shall still present: I can make the statement: "I am unique. I am as unique as my finger prints are unique. There is no other human being, ever has been or will be, who is like me." And I can make the statement: "I am you, I am the all, there is no individuality, uniqueness in me at all." If you would make the statements by saying, in some respects I am unique and in others I am not, then of course you have no truly paradoxical statement. Then this statement fits very well, as to Aristotelian logic, because you don't really contradict yourself. You say: "Here I am unique, here I am not." The statement which I am making here, is meant in the paradoxical sense. This is not so much a matter of a statement, but of experience. Do I experience myself, at the same time, and the same subject, I, as completely unique, and as completely not unique—as completely I and as completely that which I share with every human being and in some extent which I share with any living being: with a fly, or with a flower, namely, the quality of life in me? Do I experience both aspects of my life, or do I not?

Our consciousness, our awareness, is greatly influenced by Aristotelian logic. It is very difficult to experience a reality which can be experienced only in paradoxical terns. What we tend to do is to separate the two poles of the paradox, and then to feel either, we are completely unique; or to feel as the Christian mystic often felt, I am nobody, I have no individuality, I don't exists and I am completely dissolved in God or in mankind; or as a profoundly masochistic or submissive person may feel who has no sense of individuality. As soon as in any polarity we separate the two poles, the same happens—if I may use a simple analogy—if you have a positive and negative pole of electricity. If they are at a certain distance, you will have a spark. If you separate them completely, there is no spark, and if the distance disappears there is no spark either, the current will just flow through.

I do believe that with regard to the basic facts of life, we have to live on the paradox, and *we have to think in the paradox, if we want to understand life.*

Another example where we deal with a paradox too is the factor of time in analysis. Actually I can say, you or I can wake up, can break through the defenses, any minute, right now, and I can say it may take years. Experientially, there is a paradoxical attitude, namely that I expect it can happen right now, and that I expect it will take years. But if you separate the two poles, then if you assumes logically, it will take many years, then you don't expect it may happen right now. If on the other hand, you are convinced it will happen right now, you will be terribly disappointed tomorrow if it hasn't happened. From the whole literature, and I am sure there are other examples, I can give only an example for this paradox from the Talmudic literature, about the expectation of the Messiah. The Jews in their tradition expected the Messiah to come any moment, come right now. At the same time, the Talmud had a very strict and rather urgent message about it: One doesn't push the Messiah, one should not be impatient. There is a concept of patient-impatience, namely of a paradoxical patience, in which you are prepared every moment, and yet at the same time in which you may also expect it may happen in years or in the life of mankind; it may happen or take thousands of years.

The question is of the inner experience: of being able to feel both attitudes at the same time, and in spite of the fact that they are contradictory. Also the next example has to do with the attitude toward the patient: For any person whom one really understands or tries to understand, one has a feeling of responsibility for that person. I am responsible for you, because once I come close enough to you, you might say: "You are my brother," and I am indeed my brother's keeper. But, at the same time, with equal truth I have to say: "I am not responsible for you at all. You are responsible for yourself; God may be responsible for yourself, your genes may be responsible for yourself, the whole universe may be responsible for you, not me." But, again, this is a paradox which one has to experience because if you tear the two sides apart, then indeed either you feel guilty and you feel an unrealistic responsibility—and in fact you can hardly help anybody, you will only harm him—if you only feel the responsibility; if you feel only the irresponsibility, then indeed you are indifferent and cannot help either. The attitude I am talking about is again to live on the paradox that both statements—I am responsible, I am not responsible—are equally true, and I live on this and with this contradiction.

I could give many more examples of such paradoxes but I won't try to do that. All I want to do really is to make clear a point, which in our Western thinking is very difficult to grasp fully. It is so strange to us: the true experience of two contradictory facts, two contradictory statements, and the capacity or the willingness to live on these contradictions, and not to think that *because* they are contradictions, they cannot be true, or it cannot be real.

2. Alienation as a particular form of unconsciousness

The problem of alienation is really a continuation of the topic of repression, or of unconsciousness, or of dissociation, because alienation is perhaps the most frequent and the most characteristic form in which we in this culture, at this time, do dissociate experience. Alienation is, you might say, a particular form of dissociation, or you might even go further than that and say, all dissociation is a form of alienation. Nevertheless, I think that cannot prevent one from talking about it very seriously.

To describe the mechanism of *alienation* in psychological terms one can say: By alienation I project an experience, which potentially is in me, to an object over there.

I alienate myself from my own human experience and project this experience on something or somebody outside, and then try to get in touch with my own human being, by being in touch with the object to which I have projected my humanity. That holds for alienation and idolatry. The two terms refer exactly to the same phenomenon. The one term is used by Hegel and Marx and the other is used by the prophets of the Old Testament.

Both terms, alienation as well as idolatry, mean that I deprive myself, I empty myself, I freeze, I get rid of a living experience. My own thinking, my own loving, my own feeling is projected onto a person or thing outside. I can get it back by the relationship to this thing, which has become the representative of that which I have deprived myself of. I abdicate so to speak certain human powers, put them on the emperor, on the pope, or whatever it may be, and from now on, this figure *there* represents me, but I am bound to him, because if I am not close to him, I am lost, because, if you please, he has my soul. In Goethe's *Faust* Mephisto, as long as he is important for Faust, really has his soul. He has part of him, but Faust gets away from him and comes on his own.

The prophets of the Old Testament have expressed in many ways, what they call *idolatry*. In the concept of idolatry, of course we do not deal with the question whether there is one God or many Gods. For the prophets of the Old Testament, idolatry is that man worships the work of his own hand and bows down to things. In this process man becomes a thing himself. In this process, he limits himself, reifies himself, kills himself, because he becomes dependent on things towards which he has projected his human powers, but which are now in the hands of the saints.

These "things" can be idols; as you read it in the prophets, one time, a man takes a piece of wood, one half he makes a fire and bakes his cake and with the other half, he makes a sculpture and worships it as his God. Or, it can be a state, or a powerful institution. It can be anything. What is in common is always the fact that man abdicates his own creative powers and is in touch with them only indirectly by submitting to the idol, by worshipping the idol.

Marx more than anyone else has clarified the concept of alienation. Actually alienation is in the center of his system and particularly in his main works it is clear. In the *Economic-philosophical Manuscripts* (1844) he says: "The object produced by labor, its product, now stands opposed to it as an *alien being*, as a *power independent* of the producer." (MEGA I, 3, p. 83; quoted in E. Fromm, 1961b, p. 95.) If you read the prophetic description of the idol, you will see that it is almost literally the same description. And in order to deepen Marx's concept of alienation I quote from the *German Ideology* (MEGA I, 5, p. 22; quoted in E. Fromm, 1961b, p. 52f.): "This consolidation of what we ourselves produce, which turns into an objective power above us, growing out of our control, thwarting our expectations, bringing to naught our calculations, is one of the chief factors in historical development up to now."

If you really listen to Marx's words then you are forced to think of the atomic bomb, because that indeed is that "consolidation of what we ourselves produce, which turns into an objective power above us, growing out of our control, thwarting our expectations, bringing to naught our calculations," and indeed it threatens to do so.

Today the *bureaucracy* is an idol to which we project our own will, tomorrow it may be an electronic computer, because a bureaucracy is only, you might say, an imperfect step to what an electronic computer can do much better and much more correctly. You feed data, the data are collected, processed and given a certain principle and you come out with what sounds like a decision. It is a logical consequence of certain data, processed under certain premises.

If you speak today with the average person, let us say, about the danger of war, he will say: "This is all too difficult for me, I don't know." Not only the average person, many persons who ought to know, will say: "I don't know, they over there will make the decisions." The average person has stopped to think, has projected his power of thinking and willing on a bureaucracy over there and is in touch with his own human quality of willing and thinking only inasmuch as he worships this bureaucracy. The bureaucracy is an idol of decision.

God today is an idol of love and wisdom. People are not loving, and they are not wise, but since it is difficult for man to live completely without love and wisdom, they go to churches and worship God. Since they have projected love and wisdom on to God, they are once a week in the company of their own love and wisdom, by being in the church, or by using the name of God. At least they feel they have not completely lost love and wisdom, but they are alienated from it; it's not their own anymore, it is that which they get back from God. It's not an experience, but an indirect being-in-touch-with that which they have already lost, but not given up.

The *hero* is an idol of courage. I have no courage, but if I identify with the hero and worship the hero, I am in touch with whatever courage I might have.

Words in general and *thoughts*, become the generalized idols. They substitute for experience. Needless to say, that we have here a most ambiguous phenomenon. Actually if you say a word, by saying the word, you alienate yourself already from the experience. The experience is really there only, just a moment before you say the word. Once the word is said, it's already over there. But, at the same time, of courses the same was true with an abstraction, the same holds true for a concept. But it is obvious that this is also a process of increasing differentiation, of increasing thought. We deal here again with a paradoxical problem, that you speak the word to express something and the moment you have spoken it, you have already killed what you were expressing. The ambiguity of "words," the ambiguity of "concepts," and yet all that matters is really where the word comes from. If you say a word which comes from your experience, then the word will remain in the living context in which it is spoken an expression of the experience. If you speak a word which comes from your brain and yet which according to its contents should came from experience, then indeed your word is empty and is nothing but an idol, a little idol.

Let me mention a few instances in which this problem of alienation is particularly significant from the standpoint of what we go through in *psychoanalysis*. By, "we go through," I mean both being analyzed or analyzing somebody.

Take, for instance, *transference*. Of course, one can look at transference from the standpoint in which Freud looked at it, a repetition of the infantile image of the parents. That is in a sense perfectly true. But I would say there is one difference between the love of the child for the mother, and the transference for the analyst in the figure of the mother, because the child still loves the mother in an unalienated way. It *really* loves the mother. The mother means her milk, her nipple, her skin, her smile, her arm, but this is not alienated experience. But what happens in the transference situation? Especially in the very violent transferences, I impoverish myself, even more than I was before I went to that analyst, because now I have found an idol. I project being desperate about my own powers, being desperate about my own strength. I project all I have got, or all that I have left to the person of the analyst and then trying to get in touch with all my human richness by the intouchness with the analyst.

You may call it by submission, by the love, or whatever it is, but actually it is the same process as an idolatry: that emptying oneself is a condition of complete submission-dependency because now I have even ceased to exist authentically. I have now become completely dependent on the idol. This becomes a matter of being or not being, because I lose myself completely if the idol leaves me. This can happen in more extreme forms, this can happen in milder forms. I don't mean that what I am saying here about transference being in contrast to the theory of Freud or many other people. The two concepts don't exclude each other at all, or don't even contradict each other. This is one aspect, as I see it, of the transference situation.

Another example of alienation that happens in many patients, or in many of us one might call the *idolatry of the self image*. There is the self image of grandiosity: He is the hero, he is the genius. Or there is the self image of the terribly modest, kind, good person. Or there are any number of self images. Actually what happens is, that the self image becomes the idol to whom he serves. That is to say, he puts in front of himself this little statue, call it modesty, goodness, wisdom, intelligence, brilliance, anything; or surliness, or even cruelty, because that is also self image. Or in some patients, simply the phallic worship.

I am referring to the subtle process in which his own self image is an idol. He transfers whatever is alive in him to the idol and now lives reflectively in terms of the idol. That is to say, that he acts not genuinely anymore, but he acts as his own idol makes him to act. You see a person who is quite consistent in his actions and yet he is frightened because his action lacks authenticity. He has emptied himself, erected the idol of the self image, lives according to this idol but he's never himself, and that's why he is frightened.

Obviously in analysis, it's terribly important to understand not only the self image but understand the mechanism of alienation or idolatry toward the self image. Actually you find quite frequently that this self image is built up as an escape from a negative self image. You find the boy, let us say, who by his father and mother, or God knows by what circumstances, has been impressed by his own worthlessness, badness. He has a self image which is not only worth anything, but "I am dead, I'm unbearable, I'm objectionable, I'm unaccepted." This self image, if he would keep it, would practically lead to destruction, because he would really worship the Moloch, to whom one sacrificed one's children. Thus he runs away from this negative self image, to a self image which he may steal from somebody. He chooses the analyst, he chooses god knows whom as his little idol in the flight from the unbearable self image which he had developed originally. He is forced to worship the idol of the self image, because otherwise he feels always in danger that he will be driven out and he will be confronted with the original negative self image, the original feeling of utter worthlessness.

Another problem is the *idolatry of thought*. A person talks and believes that his experience is in the word, and is not aware anymore that the experience is not in him, that the word or the thought has become the little idol. Using words give the impression as if I were in touch with what the word means, when I have in fact emptied myself from the experience, and am in touch with it only indirectly by being in touch with the word which is supposed to represent the experience.

Another example for alienation is the *fanatic*. Maybe I can take Arthur Koestler's *Darkness at Noon* (1940) as an example. There you have a higher functionary of the Communist Party, who has been in the Party for many years, who has been a quite decent human being. (By decent I do not mean saintly, or something of the kind, some normal human feelings toward other people.) In the process of being a high functionary of the Party, he had actually to kill more and more all that is human in him. Eventually, all humanity in this man is killed. He feels nothing anymore, he couldn't.

It happens that the Party becomes to him the idol of all that is human. The Party represents human kindness, solidarity, brotherliness, hope, love—everything. He must become the slave of the Party, because having emptied himself of all human quality he would became insane, he would lose his human identity were it not for the fact that by submission to the Party, he remains in touch with qualities which were originally his. Then comes the particular quality for the fanatic, and that holds for only the fanatic: By making these qualities into an idol and forming them into something absolute, by the complete submission to this idol, he experiences a kind of strange, fiery passion. Or maybe I shouldn't say "fiery" passion, I should say "cold" passion.

If you love, if you see, if you hear, if you enjoy, there is excitement, there is intensity connected with a real experience. The fanatic has an intensity which is not connected with what an experience pretends to be, namely, the love for mankind, freedom or whatever it may be. But this excitement is the excitement of the complete submission under the absolute. Here you have a paradox which Koestler expressed very well in the paradoxical title *Darkness at Noon.* If I were to choose a symbol, I would choose burning ice. That is to say, there is a burning in the fanatic, but at the same time everything is completely frozen, the ice burns; he is frozen, he has emptied himself completely, he has projected completely all that is human to the idol that may be his, this hate, or this nationalism, or antisemitism, or God knows what. It doesn't make any difference. But, he experiences the intensity of the complete submission and thereby being in touch with what to him is absolute humanity. Of course, one can do that with God, too, provided God is an idol. It is important to understand the psychology of the fanatic from the standpoint of the alienation and the subsequent idolatry.

Another example is *mourning*. There is a type of depressive mourning in which the dead person, or even my own dead self becomes an idol, that all that is good is transferred to that idol, and I remain alive only in relation to my connection with the dead, either with the other person who is dead, or my own dead self.

One of the most important clinically concepts, which has also to do with alienation is the *alienation of the self.* In regard to the concept of the self—the image that the self has about himself I should differentiate between two concepts: between the *self* and the *ego*. What do I mean by the experience of one's self as an ego? I mean exactly the alienated experience which I have been talking about, and which you find in so many, if not in most people today. The alienated person looks at himself as he would look at an outsider: I have an image of myself. I don't to stress here whether our image is right or wrong, but that we see ourselves as a package and from the outside.

When we think "I," we really experience ourselves as we

experience another person, although we shouldn't experience another person that way either. We experience ourselves as a thing which has so many qualities. And then you have the kind of ruminating which you find in a person: "After all, I'm intelligent," or "I'm pretty," or "I'm kind," or "I'm courageous" and so on. Actually, this is only the description of that thing over there. This ego concept is an alienated concept of the image I have of myself as a thing which I carry through in life and with which I want to do something in life.

The concept of self, as I see it, is the experience of my self as "I" in the process of being the subject of my action. By "action" I don't mean primarily that I do this or that, but in the process of being the subject of my human experience. *I* feel, *I* think, *I* taste, *I* hear, *I* love. And there are many more things, which are all the range, all the expression of human faculties. If I am not synthetic, but the authentic subject of my activities, then indeed, I experience myself in the moment of being active as the one who acts. But I do not experience myself as the ego.

The one who experiences his self as an ego experiences only his package. He looks from the outside and asks: "How have you done it?" or: "How will you do it?" By asking himself: "How will you do it?" he asks himself: "What will be the impression this little package makes on the world, what will be the price tag, if you please?" To that same extent, of course, I'm inhibited in being, in experiencing myself as a subject of my *powers*. And on the other hand, to the same extent to which I experience myself as the subject of my powers, I do not contemplate my ego. That is actually what the New Testament means as far as I understand, "slay yourself," or what the Zen Buddhists mean when they say "empty yourself". It doesn't mean "slay yourself." This slaying yourself means simply forget about your ego, because this attempt to hold onto your ego, to look at yourself from what some people call the objective standpoint, actually stands in your way of being. The experience of "I" or of "self" exists only in the process of being, in the process of relating, in the process of using any kind of human power.

I can explain the other person as another ego, as another thing, and then look at him as I look at my car, my house, my neurosis, whatever it may be. Or I can relate myself to this other person in the sense of being him, in the sense of experiencing, feeling this other person. Then I don't think about myself, then my ego doesn't stand in my way. But something entirely different happens. There is what I call a *central relatedness* between me and him. He is not a thing over there which I look at, but he confronts me fully and I confront him fully, and there in fact is no way of escape.

I wanted to mention this here as one of the most important psychological or clinical instances of alienation because you can see why this is alienation: As soon as I experience myself as that nice, intelligent doctor, whatever he may be, married with two kids, and so on, I don't experience anything. I put my experience in that image I assume. Because the image is that of the kind, nice, intelligent doctor, I am kind, nice and intelligent.

I have talked about the problem of alienation as a particular form of unconsciousness, namely the unawareness of inner experience and the pseudo-awareness of experience in the alienated person who deceives himself about experiencing when actually he's in touch with thought, in touch with the idol, and so on.

There is what you might call an original anxiety which exists in the experience of separation. We have to overcome this primary anxiety which exists usually not manifestly but potentially, by compensating for this isolation in various ways in which we overcome it. If I say "compensating" I really mean only the regressive ways because if we take the progressive way, as I see it, namely the full development of human powers in overcoming alienation, there is no more compensation. If a person has really waked up—if a person has really seen the reality of his self, has thrown away most of his ego, then indeed there is no need to compensate for anxiety anymore, because there isn't any.

If I say, there isn't any anxiety, I don't speak of personal experience because I haven't been enlightened and I have gone through a lot of anxiety, less now than I used to, so please don't feel as if I were talking here by saying that's all very simple, and I am talking about something I know. But I do know enough and I have known a few people who hadn't any anxiety, not because they had repressed anxiety, but because they had solved the problems of their lives. These people have been very important for me as models, if you please, to see what's possible. I doubt whether I ever will achieve it, and I don't speak in this sense, but nevertheless what matters is how far one goes.

Doctor Suzuki once made a remark which I think is quite pertinent also to analytic work. He said: "Take a room which is completely dark, that is to say, absolute darkness, no light. As soon as you bring one candle into this room, the situation is totally changed. Before that candle came, there was absolute darkness, and when this candle comes, there is light. Now, then you bring ten candles, and a hundred candles, and a thousand candles, and a hundred thousand candles, and the room gets lighter and lighter and lighter. . . . That makes a great deal of difference. And yet the decisive event has happened when the darkness was broken by the first candle." I think personally of human development in terms of an increasing light. What I think it is important to bring the first candle into one's own life, or into the life of the patient, if one can.

I differentiate between what I call here the basic or primary anxiety, from the secondary anxiety by which I mean simply the anxiety which is aroused when one of the compensatory mechanisms is affected. To give an example: If a person has compensated for his anxiety by the image of himself as the successful man who is always successful. But one time he's a failure—bang. Then the compensation doesn't work anymore and then the original anxiety comes out, but not in reference to the original problem—that of separateness but in reference to the problem of the compensatory mechanism.

As long as you share your defects, that is to say, your pathology, your inability to be fully developed, to be productive—as long as you share it with the group, usually you do not have a manifest neurosis. Because you have the very reassuring and very important feeling: "I am like the rest, I am not isolated, I'm not sticking out.... I am not alone, I'm not separate." While, if you happen to have a kind of problem which does separate you, which is not the usual manifestation, very often because you are the more sensitive person, because your individuality has not been rubbed out so drastically, because you haven't been so smudged—then, indeed, you feel yourself isolated, and then you produce out of anxiety certain symptoms which we call neurotic symptoms. This is the problem of all neurotic symptoms, the non-adaptation to society by the person who suffers from a certain crippledness. I am aware that there are many complex factors in it. But what I do mean to say is that I think we must differentiate between the fact of crippledness, that is to say, of the narrowing down, impoverishment of human faculties, of aliveness, from the fact of manifest symptoms, and that this makes a great deal of difference.

3. Implications for being related to the patient

The aim of the analytic process is to help a patient grasp his hidden total experience. I emphasize obviously the "hidden" experience, but also the "total" experience, because I do not think the understanding of partial, small, isolated aspects of that which is hidden is enough for more than symptomatic cure. I think for the cure of symptoms indeed very often, the understanding of the isolated hidden or repressed experience which leads to that symptom formation will be enough. For the change of character I think the aim of analysis can only be to grasp the hidden "total" experience. That is to say, I cease to be a thing, I cease to be a stranger to myself, and I begin to experience what I am—to experience what I really feel, what I really experience. Obviously from this follows a few statements of what analysis is not.

a) How we should not be related to the patient

(1) Psychoanalysis is *not a historical research into the past* of a person. Historical research in the past is important only inasmuch as it makes it easier for the patient by having certain memories, by renewing or by reliving certain feelings of his childhood, to be able to experience that which is now repressed, which is now away from him, namely something he feels now. So one must always protect oneself from letting analysis deteriorate. It has value only when it's a part of uncovering what is the hidden experience the patient has now.

(2) Psychoanalysis is also not a study of childhood patterns and learning from it in order to manage the world better now. To give a well-known example: You were afraid of your father, that's why you are afraid of authority, and when you meet your boss, then think of it that after all, you are afraid of him because you

were afraid of your father, and this will help you. This is about the same as, let us say, saying to a hypochondriacal patient, who is in a panic when he has a cold or this or that little symptom. For the first time he comes to a doctor, and the doctor tells him: "Look here, you are a hypochondriacal person, every little thing causes you this anxiety, so when you have the next time a cold and you think you have tuberculosis, remember this is a mechanism of a hypochondriacal person." That's very relieving and it's very good. I'm not criticizing it, only saying one should not spend years to drill that into the patient. He can learn it quicker, it's important, it's useful, it's helpful, but it's not analysis.

(3) I also do not consider it analysis what happens sometimes explicitly or implicitly, as if psychoanalysis were a kind of teaching a patient the skill of living. That takes a wise man to do that, and I'm sure sometimes you find such a wise man who can teach the skill of living. It's very important and very helpful, but it is not what our profession is. We are not counsellors of wisdom. We promise something very specific: We are specialists in the understanding of the unconscious, that is to say in helping the patient in experiencing dissociated material. And we promise furthermore that there is a reasonable chance that if we do that the patient may feel better.

I think we have to live up to this promise, because otherwise I do not think we have any right or claim to call us psychoanalysts. Sometimes we may give the patients a piece of our wisdom if it is there—that can never do any harm. Sometimes we may explain to him or her some simple facts of life. But if we do so, we should say so, and say: "Now, look here, I want to give you a piece of my wisdom," or: "I want to explain to you a fact of life." But we shouldn't do it in a disguised analytic form as if we were giving an interpretation. But while all this is very useful sometimes, I think the essential thing is that we must make the decision of what psychoanalysis is: Is the essential the help for the patient in uncovering his dissociated material or isn't it?

b) Premises for understanding the patient

Analysis is—to use a traditional formula—the understanding of the unconscious of the patient. That's the formula since Freud's day, and I would still say that's a very correct, good formula. That's what we are for—to understand. I would rather not use the word "unconscious" of the patient. I would rather say: to understand the patient better than he understands himself; to understand that experience in him, which exists in him, which is there and yet it has not come to his own awareness, it's obscured from him, it's separated from him.

This leads us to the question: How do we understand another person? If you have a person, in this case a person called patient, who is like me, I understand him, provided I understand myself. If I don't understand myself I won't even understand a person who is very much like me. But let us assume for a moment I understand myself, that is to say I know myself, I am aware of the reality inside of me. Thus I would understand the other person very much like me. But we don't make selections of patients in that way, and we can't. So how do we understand a person who is entirely different? How do we understand a person whose temperament is different, who is this, that and the other way? I don't have to describe to you how different people are. I think there's one answer: it is all in us.

I'm using again the same broad and rather unscientific formulation. What I mean is, *everything is in us*—there is no experience which another human being has which is not also an experience which we are capable of having. There is no string, if the other person was a violin with not four, but with a hundred strings which, when vibrating, does not touch the same string in ourselves. The only difference is—and there my example of the strings becomes pointless—that in one person this is stronger, in another person that is stronger. But if I try to understand a criminal, a man who has murdered and stolen, I can only understand him, if I become aware of the criminal impulses in me in which I could murder or steal. It's true, I'm not a criminal, so I assume in him these impulses are much stronger, they are uncontrolled, and so on. But they are in me.

This is really saying essentially what Freud had said. But I would say it's not only with regard to our bad things; if I want to understand a saintly man, a good person, I can only understand him also if this good person is in me. If a person had nothing human in him, that is to say if there is not an impulse of goodness, of kindness, of love, of health, then indeed I would say he has ceased to be a human being. There is nothing in the other person which is not also in me. That is the only basis why we can understand any other human being, especially the being who is very different, or the being who is very sick, provided we are not so sick. If we are also sick, we sometimes understand better certain things.

This is one premise as I see it for understanding anyone. But secondly, the question is: What do we mean by "understanding?" For instance, Edward Glover wrote in a book (1955) that actually the psychoanalyst does not know anybody else any better than any layman before he has been on the couch and has had all the thing of free association. He claims that intuitively, immediately, directly, we have no knowledge, and the only knowledge we have is through the laboratory experiment of having the person on the couch and then getting the associations. Of course, that is a way of understanding and of academic psychology, as it is the way of the natural sciences.

But I believe in this way we do not understand, really. We talk about a person; we remain outside in the same way in which I was describing before, we remain outside of ourselves. We can talk endlessly about ourselves: "I'm this and I'm that, I'm hostile, I'm not hostile, I'm masochistic, and what not" and yet we remain at the level of talking *about* ourselves. I believe, and this is a belief to which I have come over the years, more and more, that indeed we understand a person fully only as much as we are *centrally related* to him.

If we really understand the patient then indeed we experience in ourselves everything the patient tells us, his fantasies, whether psychotic or criminal or childish. We understand only if they strike that chord within ourselves. That's why we can talk with authority to the patient, because we are not talking about him anymore, we are talking about our own experience which has been made manifest through his telling us what he experiences. This is indeed where the patient analyzes us. I don't mean he analyzes us by saying anything, although that sometimes happens too—and I must say that I have learned some of the most important things from what some patients have said about me in analysis. I am not talking about that part.

If you relate to the patient not as a thing over there whom you study, but if you try to experience in yourself what a patient feels, then indeed you experience the whole realm, the whole world of that which is not in the conscious mind, and by being in touch with it, indeed you analyze yourself because you become more and more aware. I would say this is the unique thing about the psychoanalytic profession which I don't see quite in any other—that in curing the patient, we cure ourselves.

Provided we start out with this kind of relatedness and we start out after our analysis is finished successfully, we start out with a readiness to see. I would define a successfully finished analysis as one in which one can begin to analyze oneself. Increasingly one becomes aware of oneself, that means in other words the resistance is broken down to a point that one can go on by oneself. But I think the patients are a tremendous help because they just hit you over the head, again and again and again, with things which are in yourself.

Some analysts react to that with a feeling of guilt. They feel: "For heaven's sake, we are treating people, and I'm much sicker than they are," which is a kind of self-discouraging reaction. But there's also a different reaction, to say: "For Heaven's sake—so I have seen something new again—this is me." If one really, instead of running away from it and feeling guilty, permits oneself to feel that, I think one has made considerable progress.

c) Being *centrally* related to the patient

I want now to speak more specifically about the most difficult of all these things to put into words—what I call *central relatedness.* In the first place, I have to say I don't think I can explain it. It can be put into words because either you experience it or you don't. Just as little as you can really put into words what is the difference between experiencing my "I" as an ego, as an object, and the experience of "I" as an active subject of my powers, in which I forget about myself, although I'm most fully myself in the process of expressing myself.

The most convincing and natural symbol for what I'm talking about is actually sexual love because in the act of sexual love, whether the man or the woman, you forget yourself. If you don't stop thinking about yourself, you are even impotent or—if it's a woman—you are even frigid. As soon as you are not in the experience and the full subject of your experience, but you become an object who thinks: "How am I doing?"—naturally then, even here on the physiological level, you are incapacitated. Actually sexual love is in this sense one of the most significant natural symbols of being related. I'm not saying that therefore two people who sleep with each other are related for that reason. This is almost a wisdom of our body only, and I'm sure there are many people whose body is quite wise and whose mind is utterly stupid. And I think there are other people whose body may not be wise and yet, who may be tremendously related to other people. In other words, I don't mean to say that there is any one-to-one relationship between sexual behavior and the general characterological pattern. I use it only in the sense of a symbol. So I would say there is no description which is adequate, there's only description of certain aspects.

When I use the word "central relatedness" I mean the relatedness from center to center instead of the relatedness from periphery to periphery. Although these are only words, I think we have some sense of what we consider central and what we consider periphery. Relatedness from center to center means to be interested: We are interested on another person, we listen attentively, we listen with interest, we think about the person, and yet the other person remains outside. In other words, we relate ourselves, think ourselves, think about the person as, quite legitimately, psychologists in the laboratory will think about the rabbit, or the chemist will think about the fluid: it's a matter of utmost interest, he is concentrated on it, and yet this is over there, I am here.

One should try to be aware of what the kind of relatedness is between lack of interest, interest and what I call the direct meeting of the other person, with regard not only to your patients, but with regard to everybody. You will find a great deal more or less of the kind of interest which corresponds to my own contact of myself as an ego: He's there, he's nice, he's intelligent, he's a little weak, he's a little strong, he's this, that and the other. But I still think *around* him. I think about him, but I do not see him fully.

The Indians and many other philosophies have a word, that is to say, "This is you."—"This is you—I don't have to describe you, I don't have to write a treatise about you—this is you. I see you as I can see about myself, this is me." If I really see another person or if I see really myself, I stop judging. I'm not saying judgment is wrong, on the contrary. I think we have to judge others and ourselves, it's a rational function. If we don't see that we are going to hell, where the hell are we going? We have to have a judgment, where we are going. What corresponds to either principle, or what corresponds to the laws of human nature? But actually this judgment as a judgment of reason. But if you really see a person, and he may be the vilest villain, you stop judging provided you see that person fully. If you see yourself whatever you are, at that point you stop feeling guilty, because you have the feeling: "This is me."

If you have the full experience of seeing the other person you really stop judging. This is what every great artist and dramatist conveys to you. The Shakespearean villain ceases to be the villain. Take, for examples, the *Merchant of Venice*: The merchant of Venice is an ugly figure, but nevertheless, the way Shakespeare has painted this merchant of Venice, he is not a villain anymore. He is he. God knows why he is he, so. God may have made him that circumstances. He is he and he is me too. And in the process of seeing him fully, where I can say: "So this is you," I am neither tolerant or judging.

It is not a matter of tolerance, it's very different. I want to emphasize this, from what is so frequent among psychologists today, to say: "Well, if I understand why he is so, I won't judge him so hard." This is all part of liberalism, where one says: "Well, so the criminal is a criminal and this was caused by circumstances, so I put him into a nicer prison." I am not speaking of tolerance here. I am speaking about an entirely different phenomenon here which doesn't exclude the other. Once at the moment when you see yourself or another person fully, you don't judge because you are just overwhelmed with the feeling, with the experience: "So that is you," and also with the experience: "And who are you to judge?" In fact, you don't even ask that question. Because in experiencing him, you experience yourself. You say: "So that's you," and you feel in some way very plainly: "And that's me too."

To be centrally related to others is something which we ought to try, and in which we can get quite a way. For me personally, for instance, Zen Buddhism has been a very effective way in overcoming an attitude of judging which comes from my own biblical background. One day I woke up and, it had completely gone. Not that I was more tolerant—it just had gone, because there was some new experience. So I'm not speaking like one who says: "Look here, that's simple." I am speaking like one who speaks from the experience of having spent many, many years in trying to learn more and more. If I see the other person—at that point what happens is not only that I stop judging but what happens is also that I have a sense of union, of sharing, of oneness which is something much stronger than being kind, being nice, this, that and the other. There's a feeling of human solidarity when two people—or even when one person—can say to the other justifiedly: "So that is you when I share this with you."

This is a tremendously important experience. I would say short of complete love, it is the most gratifying, the most wonderful, the most exhilarating experience which exists between two people. And this is one of the most important therapeutic experiences which we can give to the patient because at that moment the patient doesn't feel isolated any more. In all his neurosis, whatever his troubles are, the sense of isolation, whether he's aware of it or not, is the very crux of his suffering in one way, there are many other cruxes but this is one. At the moment when he feels I share this with him, so I can say "This is you," and I can say it not kindly and not unkindly, that this is a tremendous relief from isolation. So another person says "That is you," and he stays with me, he shares with me this.

I do have the experience increasingly in the years that once you speak from your own experience and in this kind of relatedness to the patient, that then you can say anything and the patient will not feel hurt. On the contrary, he will feel greatly relieved that there's the one man who sees him, because he knows the story all the time. We are so naive often, to think that the patient must not know this, and the patient must not know that, because he would be so shocked and God knows what. The fact is the patient knows it all the time, except he does not permit himself to have this knowledge consciously. When we say it, he is relieved because the patient can say: "For heaven's sake, I knew that always."

Freud has used the symbol of the mirror in the sense of symbolizing the detachedness of the analyst—the so-called scientific laboratory attitude. The symbol of the mirror has often been used in a different sense, namely the mirror is that which receives everything and does not keep anything. It's not a matter of whether it's right or wrong, it's just a symbolic use. I think indeed an essential factor of this kind of relatedness is that I receive everything and do not want to keep anything, to retain anything. I'm completely open to the patient. At this moment, when I speak with the patient or the patient speaks with me, there is no more important event in the world for me or for him. I am completely open to him, and all I promise him is just that: "When you come to me, I will be completely open to you, and I shall respond with all the chords in myself which are touched by the chords in yourself." That's all we can promise, and that's a promise we can keep. We cannot keep the promise that we'll cure him. We cannot keep the promise even that we will understand everything, but we can keep the promise of being completely open, and to respond.

I have to be related to the patient, not interested in him as a scientific object, but I have to be *related* to him. This is so very ambiguous, it is so kind of shallow and yet, only if one has had the experience of the difference between liking somebody, being interested in somebody, as against the full central relatedness to a person in which I feel fully: "This is you."

In this process we must forget that we are the doctor, that we are the analyst. We must forget that we are supposed to be well, and the patient is supposed to be sick. And we must not forget: this is also paradoxical. If we forget it indeed, this is too bad because our activity would be lacking in centeredness which is necessary. But at the same time, we must forget it. Because as long as I am the doctor and there is the patient, as long as I'm not relating myself to him as from one human being to the other, I am treating him like an object. As soon as I think: I am normal and he is nuts, I cannot experience the fact that we are the same, in spite of the fact that we are not, at the same time. And also, as long as I think I am curing him, I do not experience the full situation of relatedness.

Seeing the patient means to see a person as the hero of a drama, of a Shakespearean drama, or a Greek drama, or of a Balzac novel. That is to say, you see here a unique bit of life in human form which is born with certain qualities, which has struggled, and—this is remarkable—survived in this struggle with all difficulty, but which has given him specific and peculiar and individual answers to life.

To be born raises a question because of the inner dichotomy of human existence. We have to answer this question at every moment of our life, not with a thought but with our whole existence. There are only a few answers to these questions, namely the various types of regressive answers and the progressive answer. They are not so many—my hunch would be there are six or eight answers since we know anything about the human race, how to answer these questions. Each person answers the questions of life in his particular way. Of course there are, you might say, individual variations which are infinite, and which are different for every person. But at the same time there are some big categories of answers.

We have to see that each person's existence is a drama in which he or she gives successfully or unsuccessfully his or her specific answer to the problem of life. And we have to understand the total answer which he or she gives. This total answer can be the answer of complete regression to mother's womb, it can be the answer of remaining on mother's breast, it can be the answer of being bound to father's command, it can be the answer of the full development of his own powers. And not only these. There are a number of variations of them. But it's always a total structured answer, and that is why I say this is to be looked upon like the hero of a Shakespearean drama.

The answers a person gives to life are not just a little bit here a fragment, and a fragment there. It is a totality, it is always a structure, and you can understand this person only if you understand the total structure of the answer which he gives to existence: How does he try to remain sane? How does he try, and has he tried, to solve the problem of his relatedness to the world? You have to see the *total* answer which a person gives. Whether he is psychotic or neurotic, or so-called healthy, this doesn't make any difference. Every one gives an answer which is total and structure-like.

From the very beginning one should attempt to see, to understand this total answer. From the first hour, one should begin to ask oneself: "What is the prop of this drama?" and not be seduced to grab this and to grab that because one is afraid one wouldn't understand the whole. I believe every person becomes intensely interesting if one understands his drama. It's not a matter that he has to be terribly intelligent. The human drama is something exceedingly interesting provided we understand it, and don't lower the significance of a particular struggle of a person in his existence to trivialities.

d) Being aware of the own mode of relatedness

I am convinced you cannot separate your mode of relatedness to the patient, your realism as far as the patient is concerned, from your own mode of relatedness to people in general and from your realism in general. If you are naive and blind, to your friends and to the whole world, you will be exactly as naive and blind to your patients. You will pick out certain little things, where by your technical training you have learned this is this, and that is that, and yet you will not really understand the person. To really relate oneself is not a matter which depends primarily on the object, but it is a faculty, it is an orientation, it is something in me, and not something in the object. If I am caught in fiction and unreality as far as other people in general are concerned—myself, my wife, my children, my friends, the whole world—then I'm just as caught in fiction as far as the patient is concerned.

This also means that if we really want to understand the unconscious, that is to say that part which exists and which the social filter, as I call it [cf. E. Fromm, 1960a, pp. 99–106;

1962a, pp. 115–124], does not permit to come into awareness, then indeed we have to transcend the frame of reference of our society. I would put it this way: We can understand the unconscious fully only if we are critical and aware of the limitations of our own culture and the patterns of our society. If we fall for them like everybody else, then indeed we cannot really understand more than those slight differences in which the person dissociates more than, let us say, beyond the call of duty, or social duty. Then we understand an extra little bit of fear, an extra little bit of anxiety, an extra little bit of alienation, but this extra little bit which is individual is not quite enough to understand a person fully. The critical understanding and awareness of the fiction in the social pattern in which we live is a very essential condition for the full awareness of the dissociated part of another person. In addition to that I would say, that it is very necessary to understand other societies and other cultures, from the primitive ones to the civilized ones—to understand and see simply other possibilities of structures and experiences which for them were conscious but which for us are unconscious.

To give an example: In the ancestors of the Skandinavians in the early middle ages they had a secret society called the Berserker. Berserker means literally the Bear Shirts (*Bärenhemdige*). The purpose of this society was if you were initiated to transform yourself into an animal of prey, into a bear. That was saintly, that was the highest spiritual achievement: going back to the animal, becoming an animal. And the sign of this was the highest degree of rage, in which a person worked into an insane rage. But this was quite conscious, because in this insane rage he felt he had dropped all that which is human and he had become an animal and that was his original life. (It's very strange that from the Bear Shirts to the Brown Shirts is only two thousand years. Actually, if you take a man like Hitler with this particular kind of craziness, these insane rages were one of the most characteristic traits of his.)

I give the Berserker as an example, and of course we have thousands of others. If I want to understand a person with an insane rage, then indeed it helps me a great deal to know something about the Bear Shirts. Because there I can see that the insane rage is not just a peculiar individual kind of thing which is typical for this person, and I talk about the aggressiveness and destructiveness of his mother, and so on—but that this rage is an answer to life. This is a religion, it happens to be his secret, private religion. The more we know about other forms of experience outside of our own cultural frame of reference, the more we are able to understand in ourselves and in others, to experience that which in our society happens to remain outside of consciousness because it doesn't fit.

4. About the first sessions

Let me come to the question: What is the *plan of an analysis*? Does one have any plan beyond the aim of psychoanalysis: to understand the dissociated part of the patient, and to help him to understand it? I think one could do something more even in this general sense: to follow a strategic maxim. It is necessary to engage oneself, to be in it, to see the patient, to be related to him and to respond to the patient. One can see what one can do, where it leads. One cannot make a long plan before one has jumped into the situation—and "jumped" is not just to listen, to be interested, but is what I spoke of before, to see the patient, to encounter the patient if you please, to be engaged with the patient.

Aside from this very general idea, we might say the first thing one should do is *to form an idea of what this person was meant to be*, and what his neurosis has done to that person as he was meant to be. I don't mean that in a religious sense particularly or in a teleological sense. I do mean it in the sense that indeed we are not born as blank sheets of paper, we are not born even only with some of us being more timid and others of us being aggressive; I believe we are born already with a very definite personality, which by our life experience can be twisted, deformed, changed. An apple tree if it grows well, will grow good apples, but never pears. And an orange tree will grow good oranges and not apples.

The analyst should have an idea of what was this person meant to be. How would this person be if he had grown in lines of what he was meant to be? How would this person be if his development had not been distorted and neglected?—I admit that is not easy, and I don't mean to claim that one can always do this easily, or perhaps not at all. Nevertheless it should be attempted. One should never only look at the neurosis per se, and one should make the assumption which many people do make—as if all people were born more or less the same, and as if the neurosis is the deformation of the objective pattern of man which is the same for all. It isn't. The neurosis is the deformation of the particular person. Thus well-being for him means the restoration of his specific personality.

You might say here, suddenly I'm talking about the uniqueness and specificity of a person when I have been talking before about the fact that we are all the same. Well, I tried to explain that both are true. This is not a play with words, indeed we are all the same and yet we are all completely unique. If we were not all the same, I could not understand the patient, but if I think that because I understand the patient, his growth, his development would make him a person similar to me, then indeed I understand very little.

One should have a picture of the patient, and secondly *this picture of him must be based on a theory*—on a theoretical model or plan. Otherwise I'm lost because I have no frame of reference. This is a great advantage of the Freudian theory that there was a model, that there was a theory. I'm advocating that quite regardless of what your reaction is to my own theoretical frame of reference: Have one! And don't try to think you can really understand anybody profoundly unless you do it on the basis of a model of man—maybe it Freudian or anything else.

The next step is that I try to see what are the *chances for profound change*? This depends on factors like vitality, the degree to which the patient suffers, the life circumstances which further or do not further the degree of his own genuineness, his gift for honesty, the degree of his resistance. Some people are born with a tremendous gift for honesty, and other people are born with a small one. I don't mean to say that necessarily the latter ones are necessarily dishonest but it's much more difficult for them to be honest. That is to say, the circumstances have to be much more favorable for them to be honest than for the other ones. You'll find there are people that can live among thieves and murderers and they are not in danger of losing their honesty. You find another one where the margining is so small that even a slight seduction is already enough to lead him to the path of sin, if you please.—All these things you have to appreciate. And then you have to make a judgment: What are really the chances of analysis as against other efforts, namely supportive therapy, good counselling, or stopping it.

You must be very aware to make up your mind—not necessarily the first hour, or the first week, but not waiting four years until you eventually get it aware by the very simple fact that nothing has happened in four years. If you can probe, you can make remarks in which you hit something, in the second or third hour, something which you believe is essential and dissociated. You can make it in an incidental way and you can see, watch the patient's reaction: There is a flicker of recognition there—very good, if that happens by the third hour. Maybe a little smile, maybe a nod. Or, there is a violent reaction and you can judge: Has that a paranoid quality, or is it just a reaction of the kind that you can cope with it, and very well with it in the next three months? Or there is a blandness with which the patient will say: "Oh, yes, how very wise you are," but you see he has not reacted at all. If you do that five times, ten times in the first few months, and you get a pretty good feeling for what this patient can really react to and what chances are there for analytic treatment.

Another factor in this sizing is to *appreciate the resistances*: the degree of what are the main repressions and what are the main resistances. Then one decides whether this is really somebody whom one can analyze or somebody for whom one, if one wants to do anything, cannot analyze. In the latter case the method of symbolic satisfaction is indicated. The patient is really very sick, he really needs satisfaction via motherly help. The analyst gives him satisfaction in one way or another. Under this condition, the patient can go on existing. If you choose to do that, that is therapy on the base of analytic understanding, but you know also very well it's therapy which stops short of the final awakening of the patient, because he or she cannot go beyond a certain level.

In the first place psychoanalysis should begin—and I have said this not so rarely to a patient—with an honest and realistic appreciation. Not just with a phrase like this: "Of course, I can't guarantee that you will be well by the analysis." This sounds very honest, but it isn't very honest because it implies: "Of course, we can't guarantee . . ." Of course, *but* there is a reasonable expectation that we will do it. There is no such reasonable expectation.

The therapeutic success of analysis is by no means one in which one could say, aside from somebody who is terribly sick, the likelihood is that the analysis will help him. I'm not saying this as something destructive. I have great faith in psychoanalysis, and the longer I work at it, the older I am, the more so. But for heaven's sake, in this respect analysis is not different than some methods in medicine. If it is sufficiently important for a patient—in case it's a problem of his life—he will eagerly use a method which has a 10% chance or a 5% chance. But the doctor should be honest with him because otherwise he does not challenge the forces in the patient which strive for health, because he prevents the patient from seeing the seriousness of the situation.

I want now to speak about some things which I've observed from my experience with supervision and in seminars, as the *main faults which I see in students*. In the first place, I find that many young analysts, there may be some older ones, are really frightened of the patient, and have every reason to be frightened of him. Here comes a man with a problem which he has carried for forty years, it's terribly difficult, we know so little, from our experience, we know it's not the regular thing that we have learned. And this man comes in and believes that we can solve his problem. And in addition: He pays us, and quite handsomely, sometimes.

This is such a nerve, that we undertake to promise that we can help him, that naturally we are defensively frightened. I'm not saying we shouldn't undertake it, but we should be aware of what magnitude this enterprise has, how little prepared we really are for it. We are building an adventure for him and for ourselves, and that we have no reason to deceive him with an air and attitude as if this was just a matter that he comes and everything will be fine if he only comes to our office. Then we will be much less frightened of him, because we will not try to give him the impression that we are so certain.

In this respect we do not imitate the physician in general; if you come to a physician with a broken arm or with an appendicitis or something, and the physician will say: "For heaven's sake, I don't know whether I can ever cure that"—that is rather frightening to you, but you will go to somebody else. We really are not in a position in which the average physician is, but most differently, because we deal each time with a most difficult, doubtfully curable illness. But if we are aware of this and don't get ourselves into smug situation of the analyst who sits on this side of the table or the couch, we are already less frightened of the patient.

Analysts share with Protestant ministers an area in which there is an unadmitted doubt—with the ministers about God, and with the analysts about the unconscious. Officially, the ministers believe in God, otherwise they couldn't function, and officially the analyst believes in the unconscious and that the method is to uncover the unconscious. But I discovered that many analysts don't really believe in it. They pretend to, because how could they have patients, and belong to school, and graduate and so on unless they did—just as a minister has to pretend he believes in God, otherwise he would be kicked out of his congregation. Actually, there is a great deal of disbelief, doubt, double-talk, and wiggling out of this whole thing by all sorts of rationalizations.

This creates a second element which I think analysts and ministers have in common: an amazing, constant sense of guilt, (a) for deceiving oneself, because one doesn't really quite believe what one's saying; (b) in deceiving the patient because the analyst thinks secretly: "For heaven's sake, I'm much sicker than he is, and I never got better", and secondly: "This unconscious I've really never experienced, and yet I have to go on preaching all this doctrine of the unconscious and salvation by uncovering the unconscious."

I have sometimes started a seminar by simply asking the question: "Have you ever seen anybody who was cured or essentially helped by psychoanalysis?" That would be really absurd if you take a group of surgeons or internists and would ask this question. But I don't think it is absurd at all in our work, because the sad fact is that there are many of our students who have indeed never seen anyone who has been definitely changed by the uncovering of his unconscious including his own. There is a lot of self-deception, of feelings of guilt, of double-talk, but that is not analyzing. This phenomenon I think is very important to analyze.

In analyzing an psychoanalyst, one should pay a great deal of attention to his repression of all the doubts, guilt feelings, and so on, he has about the whole thing. I think he would feel it would be very helpful. Some people would really maybe do something else. Because it is a terrible burden to go on, whether one is a minister who preaches God and doesn't believe in him, or whether one is an analyst who really doesn't believe in this whole business about the unconscious. That's very unhealthy for one's mind and for one's body, and terribly boring too. So I think it's important to analyze to what extent anyone really believes in that which he professes toward his patients and for which he says he is a competent specialist.

To get out of the conflict, out of this dilemma liberal ministers talk about God, but God is only a symbol of transcendence, and many analysts find simply: "Call it psychoanalysis"—but they do counselling, they teach the wisdom of living, they give good advice, they are encouraging, they are nice. They do all sorts of things, but all that phrased in analytic words because the patient shouldn't notice that they are doing what a counsellor does.

All I'm saying here is that I find a great deal of lack of frankness in these matters within people, and a great deal of doubts and all sorts of double-talk and evasions. It is terribly important for the whole analytic profession to see this and to get out of it by putting things on the table, by clarifying it, and not by dealing with these things in a gentlemanly way that we of course all agree that we believe in the unconscious.

5. Aspects of the therapeutic process

Another thing is the *establishment of the analytic situation.* The analytic situation begins, as Sullivan has so often emphasized, with the fact that the patients are mean to analyze him and in fact that he has to demonstrate to me that he needs it. That he comes in my office for some reason or other is not enough. To establish the analytic situation it is necessary to have a situation which is as clean as a surgical room is, only in a different sense, namely it is from the very first moment on, a situation without sham and without fiction. Freud emphasized this very clearly himself. There is no word with a patient and no smile with a patient which should be or can be in this situation one of the easy, conventional, fictitious smile or words. The patient must feel when he comes here, this is another world from the one he is accustomed to, it's a world not of pretense, it's a world of complete realism in every sense. And it's a world in which the two people are related to each other in the central way, and are engaged with each other.

How can one help the patient in his task to make the

unconscious conscious, to become aware of dissociated material—to become aware of that which is in him, and yet which he doesn't dare to be aware of? In the first place one has to *avoid any kind of intellectualization*. Intellectualization is one of the greatest mistakes we make. The Freudians save themselves from this mistake by not talking. That's a good way of avoiding intellectualization. They just are silent, often for hours or for weeks. But that is no great help either. The non-Freudians do just the same, they just talk, which is not any better. So you talk about grandmother, and what happened there, and why do you feel this and so on—all sensible talk which actually only helps the patient to do what he has done all his life, intellectualize a little more his so-called problems and not to experience them. Obviously, the task of analysis is that the patient *experiences* something and not that he *thinks* more. That is so not only for an obsessional patient but for everybody, including the analyst. The function of the analyst from the very beginning of the process is to avoid on his part any kind of aid and comfort, or the tendency to intellectualize and to substitute words, ideas, concepts, for the experience.

Secondly, I think it is very important in general: *when the analyst sees something, to say it*, but to say it in full clarity. The truth has a peculiar quality, and that is, the truth since it represents reality, touches the person where the half-truth doesn't. If you are in real relatedness to another person, that is to say, really with him, in him, and you say that which is a reality in him, it is very difficult for that person to hang on to his resistances. If he is very sick, he may, indeed—I mean there is no doubt about it. But the person who is not that sick, if you are in full contact with him and say to him: "Look here, what I see is this . . .", he will usually find it very difficult to wiggle out and to give you a whole lot of rationalizations and ideas which lead to nothing.

If you tell the patient half that reality because you think he can't take it (as they say he is not ready, when in reality the one who is not ready is usually the analyst), then indeed the patient is untouched. Because the phone number doesn't ring; it's just that it has five right numbers but the sixth one doesn't ring. You don't touch it. On the contrary, the patient feels unconsciously, here you are fooled because in a way, he knows better. Here he thinks if you are so crashed and careful in formulating this, that must be terrible, you must think this is terrible. The patient gets into an atmosphere again of the same unreality and half-truth and double-talk which he's accustomed to and most people are, from childhood on, and you destroy the whole situation.

Let me give you one example which I see so often in supervision analysis. The analyst says to a person: "Well, it seems to me that you feel *as if you were* a child of five. The fact however is, that *you are* a child of five, affectively and emotionally, while intellectually and socially you are a man of forty." Now if I say to the patient: "You feel as if, or like, a child of five," I don't quite hit it. Because he *is* that. Of course, I have to add: "Indeed, you are also something else." But this "as if" or "like" already leaves a lee-way, leaves the door open. And the patient says, "Well, I don't *feel* like a child of five," and maybe he doesn't, but he is it. What I mean to say is, there is nothing good short of the most complete directness and reality in what I see in the patient. Now, mind you, I realize that there are situations and people where you have to weigh your words carefully, in cases of intense anxiety, in cases of a pre-psychotic state, and so on. But the majority of our patients are not that way.

I hear so often the discussion among students: "Well, isn't it too early," or: "Can the patient take that?" I find that usually funny. I am very happy I can say for myself, if I believe to understand something and if I have no special reason to think that this will harm the patient or that what I am saying is so foreign to the patient that he couldn't know it at all, I'm very happy to tell him so exactly what I see. I think to talk about the problem *as if* it were in general, *as if* our most important and difficult problem were when we utter our great insights, I think is rather ridiculous, because our great insights are by no means so frequent and we are very happy if we understand something.

If you really understand something of the unconscious, to put it that way, you have to make a decision. You have to make a decision, this is there in spite of common sense, in spite of common sense of the pattern of the culture, and I stick my neck out. I have come to the conviction this is there, this is what I see, in spite of the fact that all common sense evidence seems to speak against it. To give a very simple example, which we come across again and again. Let us say the patient has a mother who seems to be very nice, and everybody says she's nice, etc. According to conventional standards, she is a very nice woman. But actually, she's a murderess. I'm not saying that you are so quick to be impressed by the fact that somebody is a murderess, but at one point you are that in a particular case. Then you say: "Well, it seems to me your mother is a little aggressive sometimes." What you do is really, you don't want to take the responsibility for making the judgment, for making the decision of what you see.

In this respect many of us have the tendency to have life as comfortable as possible. A surgeon has to make a decision on the spot and sometimes a very responsible one of life and death. He can't say: "We'll wait two hours, and I'll think about it." He has to make it right here now. The analysts seem to be in a position in which they feel they don't have to exert themselves at all. Now mind you, if I say "the analysts" I am talking as an analyst and I know all of what I'm talking about from my own past. I'm doing this now for thirty years, I've gone through many failures, and there is not a single thing, a single criticism which I have made so far or which I shall make which I do not know from my own experience. I think it is dangerous to want to be comfortable enough not to risk to make a judgment which is against common sense, against conventionality, and which one thinks will make the patient very angry.

Another very important aspect of the analytic process is the *cutting through the resistance.* This is one of the things which one has to do systematically—cutting off one way of retreat after the other until the patient is driven into a corner. There he cannot run away from by now rationalizations, there he is forced to experience something—or he will stop the treatment and never come again. What sounds like such a shocking method or a cruel method if you please, is actually not so cruel at all, because I can drive the patient into a corner if I am with him, and if he knows it. If I am with him he really feels the solidity and the reality of my relatedness to him or our communication in relationship to me.

One could define analysis, (a) by telling the patient what one sees and therefore stimulating him to dare to see himself, and (b) at the same time by systematically cutting off ways of resistance, ways of retreat, until the point where the patient is confronted with himself and has to feel something or to get out.

What happens if the patient has gotten in touch with something which was dissociated? It is a sense of increased vitality, of exhilaration, of joy, and quite regardless of whether the thing was most embarrassing or not. He simply has gotten in touch with a piece of reality in him. If we have any reason to believe that the basic concept of Freud is right, namely that the uncovering of dissociated material leads to health, or frees our innate tendencies for mental health, then indeed this experience to me is a most convincing one which we see again and again in patients and in ourselves.

Once something is really touched, there is an increase in energy. We see then usually that this is like with a fog which goes and comes, that three days later the fog sets in again, and you have to work at it again, and you have again to attack the resistance. This is a process, you might call it *working through*, which takes quite some time. But actually, the symptom of an analytic discovery is never an intellectual: "Oh, that is very right, Doctor! I can see that you are right." The patient says that you are right, and then adds, if he's intelligent enough, still some more intellectual twists in the theory. He has not really achieved anything. But if he goes away with a feeling of exhilaration, of increased vitality, and if he leaves *us* with the same feeling, then we know indeed something of a true analytic nature has been done.

There is only one criterion for whether an hour is satisfactory or not, one minimum criterion: whether an hour was interesting. If an hour is boring, either for the patient or for myself, certainly it was wrong. I remember very well the hours in my transition from Freudian methods to other methods, when I was so bored that I couldn't wait to the end of the hour. I listened dutifully and I made every effort, and yet I was just waiting for when this hour would end. That was actually the reason why I felt there was something so fundamentally wrong in my way of going about it. I know my teachers were awfully bored too, because many of them fell asleep during the analysis, and I remember how shocked I was when I heard one of my teachers say at a party that he had found a new tobacco which helped him to keep from falling asleep. Another one said falling asleep wasn't bad because he had dreams about the patient and this was the best insight yet. (I fell asleep once or twice, but maybe I had a tendency to snore, so I didn't dare, really, to go very far in that. But I do remember I was terribly bored.)

Since quite a number of years, it is the greatest exception, even if I'm tired, that I'm bored. And that for me is the first criterion of judging an analytic hour, whether I'm bored or the patient is bored. If the patient is bored, it's just as bad, and in fact you can't even separate it if the patient is bored, I am bored, and *vice versa.*

BIBLIOGRAPHY

Bernard, L. L., 1924: *Instincts. A Study in Social Psychology*, New York (Henry Holt) 1924.

Brentano, L. J., 1916: *Die Anfänge des modernen Kapitalismus*, München (G. Franzscher Verlag) 1916.

Dewey, J., 1922: *Human Nature and Conduct*, New York (The Modern Library, Random House) 1922.

Duncker, H., 1930: *Über historischen Materialismus*, Berlin (Internationaler Arbeiterverlag) 1930.

Freud, S.: *The Standard Edition of the Complete Psychological Works of Sigmund Freud* (S. E.), Volumes 1–24, London 1953–1974 (The Hogarth Press):

—1905d: "Three Essays on the Theory of Sexuality," S. E. 7, pp. 123–243.

—1905e: "Fragments of an Analysis of a Case of Hysteria," S. E. 7, pp. 1–122.

—1908b: "Character and Anal Eroticism," S. E. 9, pp. 167–175.

—1918b: "From the History of an Infantile Neurosis," S. E. 17, pp. 1–122.

—1921c: "Group Psychology and the Analysis of the Ego," S. E. 18, pp. 65–143.

—1924d: "The Dissolution of the Oedipus Complex," S. E. 19, pp. 171–179.

—1925d: "An Autobiographical Study," S. E. 20, pp. 7–70.

—1930a: *Civilization and Its Discontent*, S. E. 21, pp. 57–147.

Fromm, E.:

—1930a: "The Dogma of Christ," in: *The Dogma of Christ and Other Essays on Religion, Psychology and Culture*, New York (Holt, Rinehart and Winston) 1963, pp. 3–91.

—1932a: "The Method and Function of an Analytic Social Psychology," in: *The Crisis of Psychoanalysis. Essays on Freud, Marx and Social Psychology*, New York (Holt, Rinehart and Winston) 1970, pp. 135–162.

—1932b: "Psychoanalytic Characterology and Its Relevance for Social Psychology," in: *The Crisis of Psychoanalysis. Essays on Freud, Marx and Social Psychology*, New York (Holt, Rinehart and Winston) 1970, pp. 163–189.

—1935a: "Die gesellschaftliche Bedingtheit der psychoanalytischen Therapie," in: *Zeitschrift für Sozialforschung*, Paris (Librairie Félix Alcan) Vol. IV (1935), pp. 365–397. Engl.: The Social Determinants of Psychoanalytic Theory, in: *International Forum of Psychoanalysis*, Vol. 9 (No. 3–4, October 2000) S. 149–165.

—1936a: "Sozialpsychologischer Teil," in: M. Horkheimer (Ed.), *Studien über Autorität und Familie* (Schriften des Instituts für Sozialfoschung, Vol. V), Paris (Librairie Félix Alcan) 1936, pp. 77–135.

—1941a: *Escape from Freedom*, New York (Farrar and Rinehart) 1941.

—1947a: *Man for Himself. An Inquiry into the Psychology of Ethics*, New York (Rinehart and Co.) 1947.

—1955a: *The Sane Society*, New York (Rinehart and Winston, Inc.) 1955.

—1956c: "Bases Filosóficas del Psicoanálisis", in: *Revista Psicología*, México, Band 1 (Nr. 2, 1956), S. 59–66.

—1960a: "Psychoanalysis and Zen Buddhism," in D. T. Suzuki, E. Fromm, and R. de Martino (Eds.), *Zen Buddhism and Psycboanalysis*, New York: Harper and Row), pp. 77–141.

—1961b: *Marx's Concept of Man*. With a Translation of Marx's Economic and Philosophical Manuscripts by T. B. Bottomore, New York (F. Ungar Publisher Co.) 1961.

—1973a: *The Anatomy of Human Destructiveness*, New York (Holt, Rinehart and Winston) 1973.

—1979a: *Greatness and Limitations of Freud's Thought*, New York (Harper and Row) 1980.

—1980a: *The Working Class in Weimar Germany*. A Psychological and Sociological Study, edited and introduced by Wolfgang Bonss, London (Berg Publishers) 1984.

—1989a: *The Art of Being*, New York (Continuum) 1992.

—1989b: *Das jüdische Gesetz. Zur Soziologie des Diaspora-judentums*, ed. by Rainer Funk and Bernd Sahler (Schriften aus dem Nachlaß, Volume 2), Weinheim und Basel (Beltz Verlag) 1989.

—1990a: *The Revision of Psychoanalysis*, Boulder (Westview Press) 1992.

—1991a: *The Art of Listening*, New York (Continuum) 1994.

—1991b: *Die Pathologie der Normalität. Zur Wissenschaft vom Menschen* (Schriften aus dem Nachlaß, ed. by Rainer Funk, Volume 6), Weinheim und Basel (Beltz Verlag) 1991.

Glover, E., 1955: *The Technic of Psychoanalysis*, New York (International Universities Press) 1955.

Knight Dunlap, K., 1929: "Are there any Instincts?," in: *Journal of Abnormal Psychology*, Vol. XIV, 1929.

Kuo, Z. Y.: 1921: "Giving up Instincts in Psychology," in: *Journal of Philosophy*, Vol. XVIII, 1921, pp. 645–666;

—1922: "How are our Instincts Acquired?", In: *Psychological Review*, Band XXIX, 1922.

Kraus, L., 1930: *Scholastik, Puritanismus und Kapitalismus*, München and Leipzig (Duncker und Humblot) 1930.

Marx, K.: 1971: *Die Frühschriften*, ed. by Siegfried Landshut (Kröners Taschenausgabe 209), Stuttgart (Kröner Verlag) 1971.

—MEGA: *Karl Marx und Friedrich Engels, Historisch-kritische Gesamtausgabe* (= MEGA). Werke—Schriften—Briefe, im Auftrag des Marx-Engels-Lenin-Instituts Moskau, ed. by V. Adoratskij, 1. Abteilung: Sämtliche Werke und Schriften mit Ausnahme des Kapital, quoted I, 1–6, Berlin 1932:

—MEGA I, 3: *Ökonomisch-philosophische Manuskripte aus dem Jahre 1844*

—MEGA I, 5: *Die deutsche Ideologie*

Mead, M.: 1928: *Coming of Age in Samoa*, New York (William Morrow Co) 1928.

—1930: *Growing up in New Guinea*, New York (William Morrow Co) 1930.

—1935: *Sex and Temperament*, New York (William Morrow Co) 1935.

Murphy, G., 1932: *An Historical Introduction to Modern Psychology*, New York (Harcourt, Brace) 1932.

Osborn, R., 1937: *Freud und Marx*, London (Verlag Victor Gollancz) 1937.

Reich, W., 1929: "Dialektischer Materialismus und Psychoanalyse", in: *Unter dem Banner des Marxismus*, Berlin, Vol. 3 (No. 5, 1929).

Sombart, W., 1923: *Der Bourgeois*, München/Leipzig (Duncker and Humblot) 1923.

Tawney, R. H., 1927: *Religion and the Rise of Capitalism*, London (Harcourt and Brace) 1927.

Troeltsch, E., 1919: *Die Soziallehren der christlichen Kirche*, in: Gesammelte Schriften Band I, Tübingen (C. B. J. Mohr) 1919.

Warden, C. J., 1936: *The Emergence of Human Culture*, New York 1936.

Weber, M., 1920: *Gesammelte Aufsätze zur Religionssoziologie*, Vol. I, Tübingen (J. C. B. Mohr) 1920.

Wolfe, B. D., 1937: *Portrait of Mexico*, New York, Covici (Friede Publishers) 1937).

ABOUT THE AUTHOR

Erich Fromm (1900–1980) was a bestselling psychoanalyst and social philosopher whose views about alienation, love, and sanity in society—discussed in his books such as *Escape from Freedom*, *The Art of Loving*, *The Sane Society*, and *To Have or To Be?*—helped shape the landscape of psychology in the mid-twentieth century. Fromm was born in Frankfurt, Germany, to Jewish parents, and studied at the universities of Frankfurt, Heidelberg (where in 1922 he earned his doctorate in sociology), and Munich. In the 1930s he was one of the most influential figures at the Frankfurt Institute of Social Research. In 1934, as the Nazis rose to power, he moved to the United States. He practiced psychoanalysis in both New York and Mexico City before moving to Switzerland in 1974, where he continued his work until his death.

ERICH FROMM

FROM OPEN ROAD MEDIA

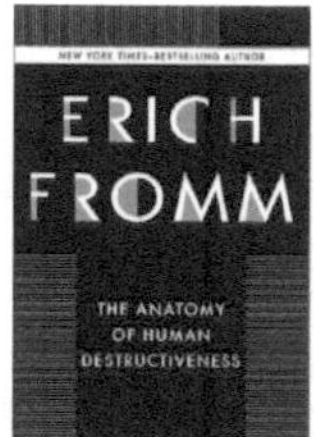

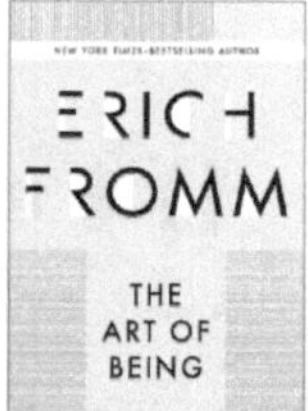

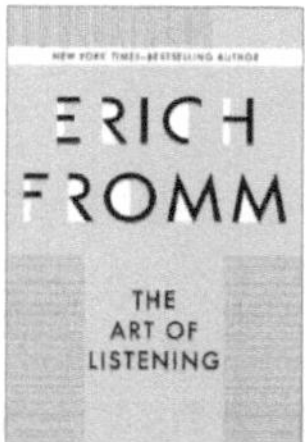

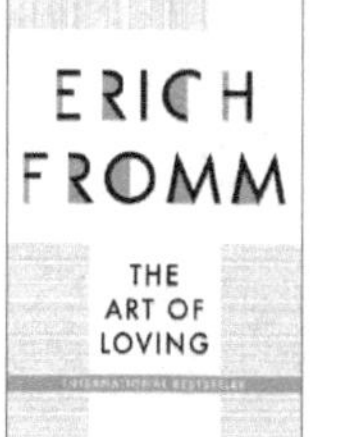

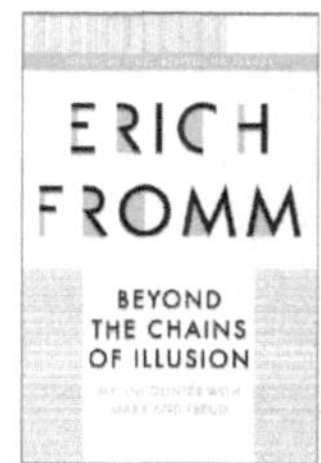

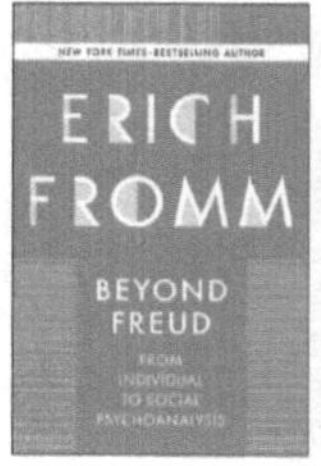

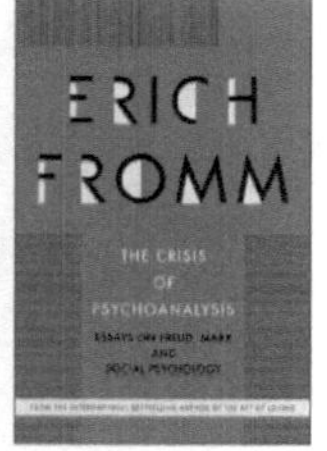

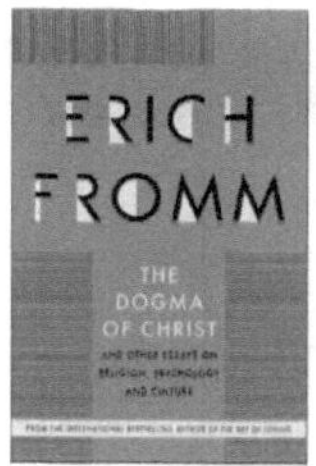

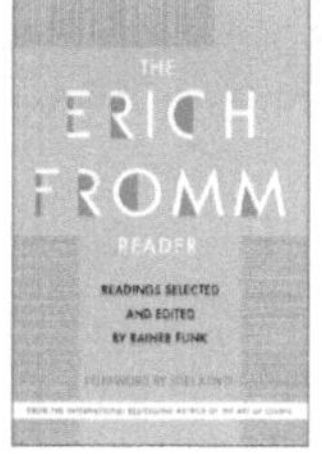

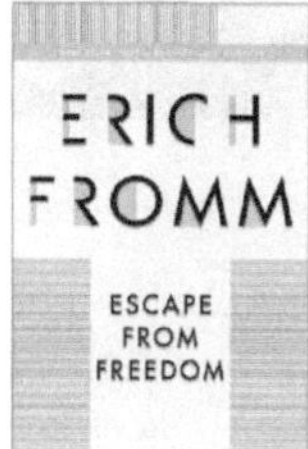

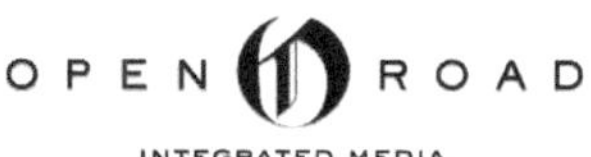

www.ingramcontent.com/pod-product-compliance
Lightning Source LLC
LaVergne TN
LVHW090612110826
845146LV00001B/356

* 9 7 9 8 3 3 7 2 0 9 1 8 0 *